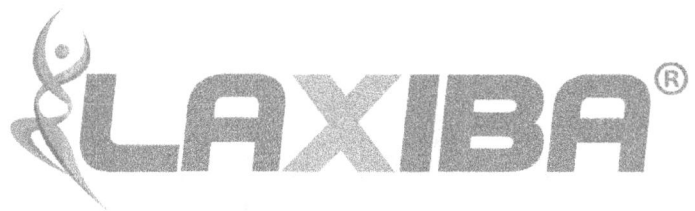

THE SORBITOL NAVIGATOR

The Standard for Sorbitol Intolerance

1. Edition

The Nutrition Navigator Books Number Four

M.Sc. J. N. Stratbucker

Laxiba
Wilmington and Koblenz

Copyright © 2016 by J. N. Stratbucker

ISBN 978-1-941978-39-9

Library of Congress Control Number 2016905805

Cover design by Mahmood Ali

Interior design by Katharina Maas and Mahmood Ali

Layout by Alexandra Krug

E-Mail of the author: John@Laxiba.com

ADP American Diet Publishing GmbH

Johannes Muller Straße 12	913 N Market Street
56068 Koblenz	Wilmington, DE, 19801
Germany	United States of America

For companies and institutions:
Are you interested in bulk orders? Visit us at: *https://laxiba.com*

The ADP American Diet Publishing GmbH holds the sales license for the book. All rights reserved. It is not allowed to use or reproduce any part of this book in any manner whatsoever. Without written permission of the author, reprints, translations, taking values or illustrations, saving it in data systems or on electronic devices as well as providing parts of the book online or on other communication services is liable to prosecution. Avoid being a cheat and only read the book, if you obtained it in a legal way.

The data set for the algorithmic ordained statements concerning sugar-alcohols is from the University of Minnesota Nutrition Coordination Center 2014 Food and Nutrient Database. The reason to acquire the database license for this book were its high quality and scope based on international research. Statements regarding fructans and galactans result from six cited international studies. Nevertheless, the contents of the book bear no guarantee. Neither the author, publisher, any cited scientist nor the University of Minnesota is liable for personal injuries or physical or financial damage. Please note that the quantities of critical ingredients in the mentioned products, which are the foundation for the stated portion sizes, are relative and in part based on derivations. The serving sizes in this book are based on approximations of various details. The precise tolerable portion size of any product varies depending on its processing, country-specific composition, degree of maturity and cultivation.

Manufactured in the United States of America

FIRST EDITION

Acknowledgments

Special thanks to M. Thor and the nutritional research team of the University of Minnesota, J. S. Barrett, J. R. Biesiekierski, P. R. Gibson, K. Liels, J. G. Muir, S. J. Shepherd, R. Rose and O. Rosella as well as the rest of the gastroenterology research team of the Monash University, all other cited scientists for their research, B. Hartmann of the Bundesministerium für Ernährung, Landwirtschaft und Verbraucherschutz, G.-W. von Rymon Lipinski of the Goethe University, and H. Zorn of the Justus Liebig University, for copyediting L. Gomes Domingues, F. Lang, C. R. Mundy, L. Popielinski, and M. Vastolo, for their feedback T. Albert, K. Bayer, U. Blendowske, D. Durchdewald, as well as my friends, especially C. Schlick and I. Kloppenburg, and all other contributors who enabled me to write this book in first place.

To my friend George Wagner for his encouragement

Contents

PREFACE _____ IX

1 INFORMATION _____ 1
   1.1 Why you deserve this book _____ 1
   1.2 Diagnostic check _____ 3
   1.3 Presentation of sorbitol _____ 6
      1.3.1 How symptoms emerge _____ 6
      1.3.2 Sorbitol characteristics _____ 10
      1.3.3 Consequences of a sorbitol intolerance _ 14
   1.4 Background of an irritable bowel _____ 16
   1.5 Abdominal discomfort in kids _____ 17

2 STRATEGY _____ 19
   2.1 A gut's change management _____ 19
      2.1.1 Signpost _____ 20
      2.1.2 Roadmap _____ 21
      2.1.3 Symptom test sheet _____ 25
      2.1.4 Keeping your balance _____ 29
   2.2 Your individual strategy _____ 32
      2.2.1 Substitute test _____ 33
      2.2.2 It depends on the total load _____ 33
   2.3 Prevalence of the intolerances _____ 34
   2.4 General diet hints _____ 35
      2.4.1 Good reasons for your persistence _____ 35
      2.4.2 Mealtimes _____ 39
      2.4.3 Eating out _____ 39
      2.4.4 Convenience foods _____ 40
      2.4.5 Medicine and oral hygiene _____ 40
      2.4.6 Nutritional supplements _____ 41
      2.4.7 Protein shakes—nutrition for athletes __ 41
      2.4.8 Fish and meat _____ 42
      2.4.9 These actions lead to lasting change ___ 42
      2.4.10 Reasons for using sorbitol _____ 46
      2.4.11 Positive aspects of the diet _____ 46
      2.4.12 Testing yourself _____ 46
      2.4.13 Sweetener's sorbitol content _____ 46
   2.5 The cheat sheet _____ 48

- 2.6 The safe products list 53
- 2.7 Recepies 57
  - 2.7.1 Kiwi sauce (e.g. with ice) 57
  - 2.7.12 Lemon bar 58
  - 2.7.2 Orange-peppermint-salad 59
  - 2.7.3 Pancakes 60
  - 2.7.4 Pizza dough 60
  - 2.7.5 Rhubarb, roasted 61
  - 2.7.6 Rhubarb cake 62
  - 2.7.7 Rucola salad 63
  - 2.7.8 Spaghetti al salmone 64
  - 2.7.9 Sweet potato- or salami & pesto-pizza 65
  - 2.7.10 Thuna pizza 66
  - 2.7.11 Tropical fruit salad 66
- 2.8 Stress management 67
- 2.9 General summary 73

FEEDBACK 76

3 FOOD TABLES 77

- 3.1 Introduction to the tables 77
  - 3.1.1 Your personal sensitivity levels 78
  - 3.1.2 Explanation of the symbols 79
  - 3.1.3 Explanation of the statements 80

CATEGORY LIST-INDEX 81

- 3.2 Athletes 83
- 3.3 Beverages 85
  - 3.3.1 Alcoholic 85
  - 3.3.2 Hot beverages 91
  - 3.3.3 Juices 95
  - 3.3.4 Other beverages 98
- 3.4 Cold dishes 101
  - 3.4.1 Bread 101
  - 3.4.2 Cereals 103
  - 3.4.3 Cold cut 106
  - 3.4.4 Dairy products 110
  - 3.4.5 Nuts and snacks 115
  - 3.4.6 Sweet pastries 118
  - 3.4.7 Sweets 123

3.5	**Warm dishes**	**128**
3.5.1	Meals	128
3.5.2	Meat and fish	133
3.5.3	Side dishes	136
3.6	**Fast food chains**	**138**
3.6.1	Burger King®	138
3.6.2	KFC®	140
3.6.3	McDonald's®	141
3.6.4	Subway®	143
3.6.5	Taco Bell®	145
3.6.6	Wendy's®	146
3.7	**Fruits and vegetables**	**147**
3.7.1	Fruit	147
3.7.2	Vegetables	152
3.8	**Ice cream**	**159**
3.9	**Ingredients**	**162**

GLOSSARY		**163**
4 ADVANCED PROCEDURES		**165**
4.1	**Level test**	**165**
4.2	**Symptom-based test process**	**182**
4.3	**Test result calculation table**	**184**
4.3.1	The efficiency check calculation table	185
4.3.2	The level test calculation table	188
SOURCES		**191**
FOOD INDEX		**207**

Preface

You just lately learned about your sorbitol sensitivity? Alternatively, are you well aware of your disease for many years? In each case, this book will help you, as it makes cooking and eating easy with its portion sizes in standard cooking measures as well as in gram and milliliter: scientifically proven and tested by readers like you. You may have tried out expensive medication or radical regimes like the FODMAP diet. Although the latter really works, it is unnecessarily strict. The aim of this book is to bring you more choice while you avoid your symptoms.

The book's information originates from intensive research and interviews with professors. The food tables in this book show you reliable serving sizes for foods concerning sorbitol. The design of the tables makes them easy to use. Moreover, they contain several specials. For example, all nine sugar-alcohols entered the portion equations to give you safer results and even products for athletes are included in the lists.

You may not have to avoid categorically all foods that contain sorbitol. It is enough to avoid eating more of them than you can stomach. By having as much choice as possible while preventing your symptoms, you increase your quality of life. How do you know how much your individual sensitivity allows you to eat? Quite simply, this book will tell you. Curious?

Then read on. In the first Chapter, you will learn about the diagnosis, backgrounds and consequences of a sorbitol intolerance. Then in Chapter 2, you discover how to implement and keep the diet. You will also find a lot of advice there concerning healthy eating in general, recipes, hints of eating-out, strategies to stay motivated to stress management. Afterward, in Chapter 3 you will find the standard portion sizes for more than 1,000 products. Chapter 4 gives you even more advanced techniques to better adapt to your sensitivity. As I deal with a sorbitol intolerance for a long time, I know about your need for clarity and practical advice. The focuses of my strategy are quality and suitability for daily use. I wholeheartedly wish you an ongoing success on your way to treat your symptoms and improve your quality of life!

Note: Despite my aim to provide the highest quality, this book should not be the sole basis for any decision you make. Talk about any diet with your doctor before you begin to limit discomfort. You are responsible for your personal health, including how you choose to interpret data and specialists' advice. I cannot guarantee you a recovery. Several causes for your symptoms are possible—to find out more get THE IBS NAVIGATOR.

1

Information

1.1 Why you deserve this book

Congratulations: You take the initiative. By buying this book, you show your will to overcome your discomforts. If you bought this book, you know that a higher well-being is not only good for you but also ever one around you. Turn your back to the symptoms-grumbler. With the proper diet, you will feel healthier and stronger and enjoy more freedom!

Learn all you need to know about your disease, reevaluate your personal story in that context and learn what you can do to live with it as best as possible. In addition, you find practical advice for a healthier diet in general on page 29 and on page 67 efficient methods to reduce stress, which often worsens your symptoms.

If you bought the book so you could learn to adapt to those in your life suffering from sorbitol intolerance, you would find out how in Chapter 2.5 and the one following it. Such behavior shows consideration for others that would make anyone glad to be a guest at your table!

That your nutrition affects your happiness is not a secret. It starts with your birth. A full and happy baby makes you happy too. The mother's milk provides the baby with the entire ingredients it needs and tolerates. As an adult, you choose the components of your nutrition yourself. Here it also holds that if you want to be satisfied, you need to eat the food your gut can handle.

Which diagnostic procedure should you have undergone? How does sorbitol affect me and how sensitive am I? How much can I eat of foods containing it without hurting myself? Which foods are free of sorbitol?

You get the answers for all of the mentioned questions. Explanations of the current scientific results and the most practical food tables for sorbitol intolerance on the market provide you with all you need to take proper action. On top of that, you find the cheat sheet for your wallet that enables you to adapt your diet even when eating out or going to the grocery store. Stop losing valuable energy to abdominal symptoms. Treat them right and start enjoying your life more in-stead; you deserve it!

1.2 Diagnostic check

Are abdominal pains, bloating, constipation, flatulence or diarrhea your ongoing companion? Without disrespect, we should find a way to get you a better spare time activity. Instead of accepting these discomforts, you should get the appropriate tools to free yourself from them as much as possible in order to spend more of your time enjoying the bright side of life.

The first thing you should do is to find out which of the potential triggers is the one that affects you. Just assuming you have a sorbitol intolerance is not enough. Going through all diagnostic procedures can take up half a year but will pay off. You will probably be able to get a handle on your symptoms and by using this book, you will also make sure to avoid unnecessary limitations concerning your diet, if you have indeed a sorbitol intolerance—otherwise get *THE IBS, THE FRUCTOSE* or *THE LACTOSE NAVIGATOR*.

To determine your profile, you should ask your local doctor to send you to an expert, a so-called gastroenterologist. Just the sound of this word might frighten your troublemakers. The specialist then first checks, whether your symptoms have a different cause than an intolerance. The diagnosis will include a **stool analysis**, an **ultrasonic check** and some camera shots inside your stomach to reject other reasons. These tests will allow the specialist to check whether there is an **abnormal bacterial colonization** of the small intestine. This migration may lead to false positives in uncovering an intolerance towards the **main triggers: fructose, fructans, galactans, lactose,** and **sorbitol**. The next test looks for **celiac disease**, sensitivity towards gluten, which is an ingredient in grains. In people who have an untreated celiac disease, the tolerance test for the cube sorbitol is often positive, even if they can stomach it if they avoid gluten-containing foods. Following this, you should take a genetic test regarding **hereditary fructose** intolerance. Hereditary fructose intolerance is rare, but it is serious: the fructose test itself can be lethal to those with this disease.

You ruled out other potential causes, and the brats are probably trembling. Great, as now they are in for: what follows are checks regarding three of the mentioned main triggers. For the so-called breath test, you will take a high dose containing fructose, lactose or sorbitol on different days. If one of these passes through to your large intestine, due to suboptimal absorption by your body, gasses emerge. The doctors measure them to find out if you have an intolerance. When the amount of gas reaches a certain level, the diagnosis is an intolerance toward the respective trigger and have to adapt your diet accordingly. The threshold for a positive diagnosis for a lactose dilution (typically containing 25–

50g) is usually 20ppm (parts per million, a concentration measure). This threshold also applies for fructose and lactose. The recommended breath test, however, is not available everywhere. In *THE IBS NAVIGATOR*, you will learn about a substitute test, in case you have no access to the breath test.

Has the breath or substitute test shown that your body has enough capacity to handle even extreme amounts of a trigger? If so, you do not need to take any further attention to that trigger; its consumption will not cause you any harm—ignore the trigger: there is no point in taking unnecessary diets. If however the test shows that you have for example an intolerance towards sorbitol, you know which of the triggers you have to render harmless by limiting your consumption of foods in which it is present.

In general, do not accept a diagnosis without a test. If none of the tests comes to a conclusive result, you have an irritable bowel syndrome that is at least—for now—undefined. Irritable bowel just means that your gut reacts sensitively to various types of irritations such as gasses inside it—more on that in Chapter 1.4. The bowel is the final segment of your alimentary canal and the section where your symptoms come to show. Irritable bowel symptoms can be defined—if you have one of the before mentioned intolerances or undefined. If it is undefined, either, you did not take a test or it showed that you do not have an intolerance to one of the mentioned triggers. Note here that no breath-test is available for fructans and galactans as of now, and you will need to test your tolerance yourself, with my *IBS* book. In both cases, the symptoms are similar, because readily fermentable carbohydrates, a group that all triggers belong to, of some sort trigger the symptoms. Incidentally, for up to 90% of patients with an irritable bowel, an intolerance to one or more of the three breath-test-triggers mentioned above causes the symptoms.

If you suffer from irritable bowel symptoms, you are not alone: 20% of Americans have an intolerance, i.e., their enzyme worker team is too small for one or more of the three triggers that one tests with a breath test. Worldwide, 10–15% of all people suffer from undefined abdominal discomfort. About 20–30% of Europeans in general, 9% of the Dutch, 22% of the English, 25% of the Japanese and 44% of West Africans are affected. Concerning children, they should only take a diet under medical supervision. By the way, a lactose intolerance can only evolve at an age above five years. All younger children can stomach lactose.

It is also possible that a doctor finds that you are intolerant according to a breath test, but you do not feel symptoms. In such a case you may still want to keep the respective diet if you suffer from depressive moods, see Chapter 1.3.3.

Summary

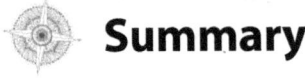

If you regularly suffer from abdominal discomfort, visit a specialist, a gastroenterologist. You may assume you have a sorbitol intolerance but only a specialist can rule out more severe diseases. Checks can take up to half a year. Many others share your fate; about 20% of Americans are affected. You are holding in your hands the key to fighting the symptoms!

1.3 Presentation of sorbitol

We depict sorbitol as cube. Why? Just imagine having a big cube in your stomach. Not a good feeling. On the other hand, a cube can have a positive effect, too. Think of a sugar cube that provides a lot of energy. Likewise, sorbitol, representin sugar-alcohols, provides you with energy, if your stomach uses it in that way.

1.3.1 How symptoms emerge

If you have an intolerance against sorbitol, your body only provides a few workers making sure your body uses the cube for energy. Few workers mean that if you eat too much of foods that contain sorbitol cubes, many remain unused by your body and arrive at your large intestine. Now, two processes are responsible for the symptoms: osmosis and fermentation. To understand osmosis, let us imagine two equal fish bowls connected by an underwater tube.

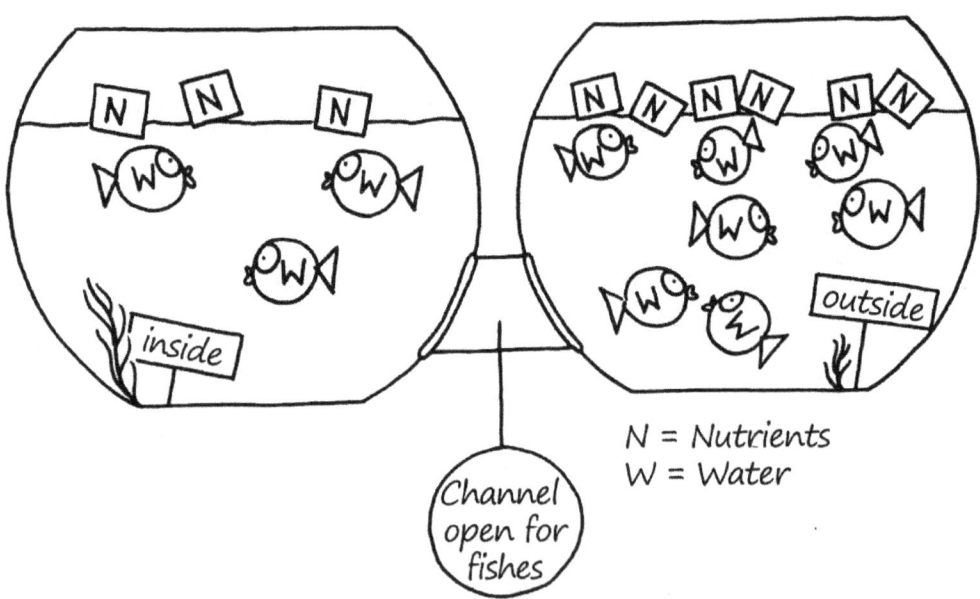

The glass on the left represents the inside of the bowel and the one on the right for the outside of it. The fishes represent water (W), and their food are either nutrient (N) or sorbitol cubes that arrive at the inside of the bowel (S). The channel enables fishes to switch between the bowls. Thus, they always swim to the glass that contains more food. Usually, this would be the outside of the intestine. Thereby, the body detracts the water from the foods—which is a good.

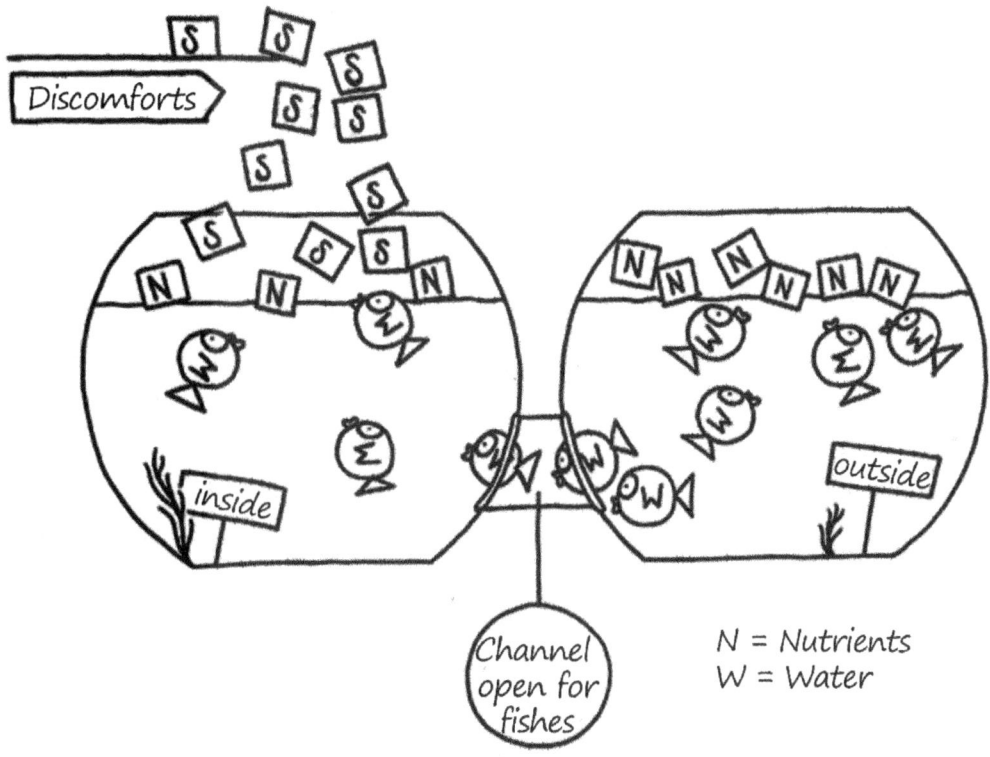

However, if you eat more of foods containing sorbitol than your enzyme workers can handle, sorbitol cubes arrive at the inside of the bowel. Hence, suddenly there is more food in the left fish bowl.

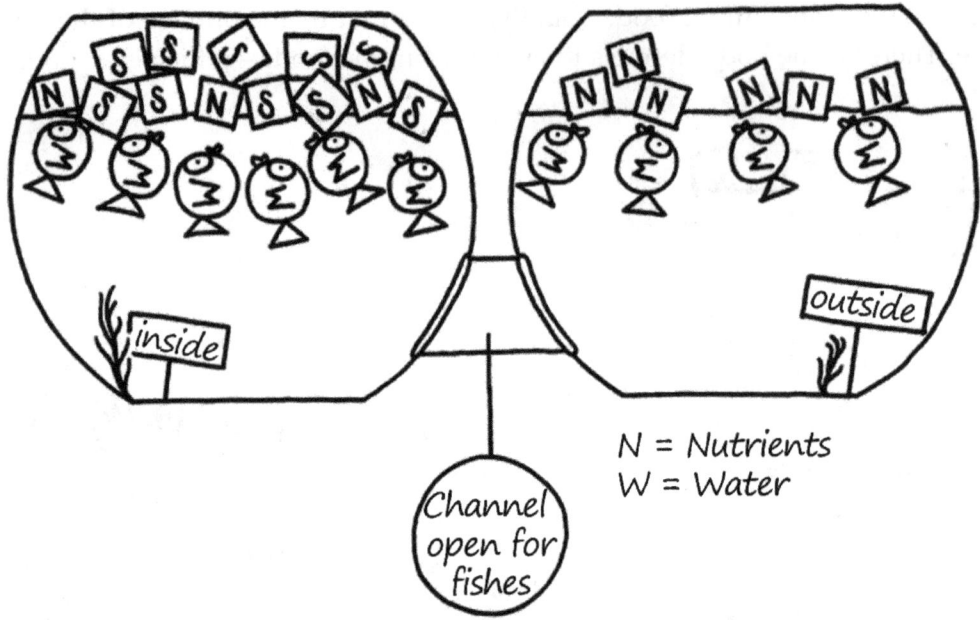

As the intestinal wall, here represented by the channel, is only partially permeable, the fishes can swim through it, unlike the food. Therefore, some fishes now switch sides and scrimmage on the left. Their movement to the left means that with the cubes water arrives inside the intestine and you suffer from diarrhea.

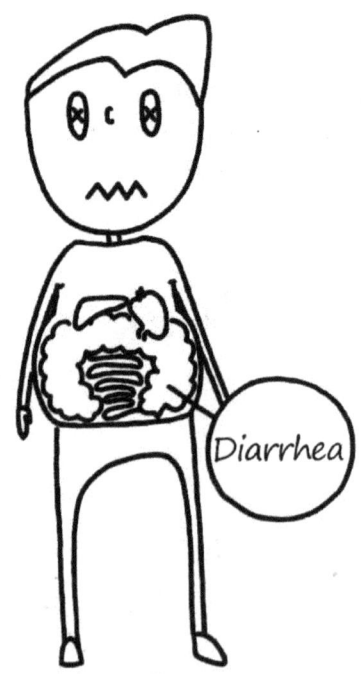

Now you know about osmosis. What causes fermentation?
As you know, you have bacteria inside your bowel, which is normal and that way for any healthy person. The issue is that these bacteria love sweets. Hence, if a trigger cube arrives at the large intestine, they do not falter and immediately consume it to help themselves to some energy.

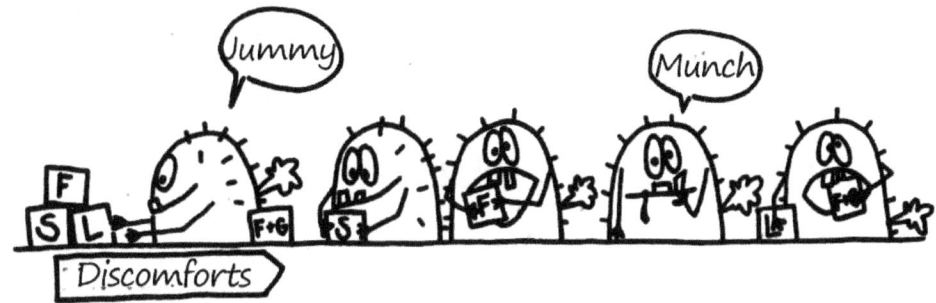

Unfortunately, though, the bacteria are less efficient at consuming the sorbitol cubes than our body is. When bacteria use sorbitol cubes, gas emerges.

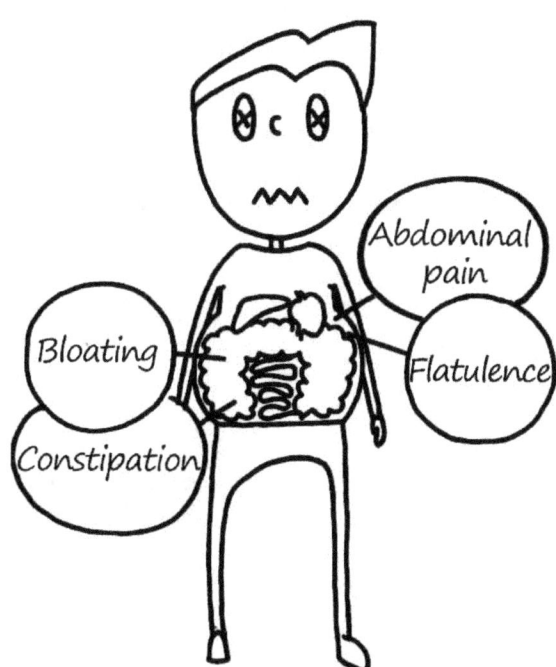

The gas either leaves as bloating or amounts and causes an uncomfortable flatulence. If the pressure increases in some regions of the intestines, this can cause deposits—constipation. If the gas enters the small intestine, it causes, even more, turmoil: it hinders some of the body's cube workers from doing their job. That is because the workers mainly sit on the gut wall and the gas reduces its contact to the stool. However, what about the treatment with a diet? In general, it is important for your health to have a diverse diet. The FODMAP approach, which you may have heard of, aims at reducing the fermentation and osmosis by lowering the consumption of all potential triggers at once. With the sorbitol standard treatment of this book, you take a more precise aim to give you more freedom concerning your food choice. With it, you only avoid sorbitol, as described in the diagnosis check. First, you should get to know it, though.

1.3.2 Sorbitol characteristics

Sorbitol is one of nine sugar-alcohols that causes symptoms in case of a sorbitol intolerance. As sorbitol is the most popular of the group, though, the label sorbitol intolerance has enforced itself. To make the text more readable, sorbitol refers to all nine sugar-alcohols in this book. Some fruits and vegetables naturally contain sorbitol. Furthermore, sugar-alcohols are sweeteners and carriers for some medicines. Diabetic products like jelly contain up to 12g per portion and chocolate up to 40g per four pieces. Moreover, sorbitol is sometimes included in ice cream, juices, oral hygiene products, sauces, sugar-free chewing gum (up to 2.5 g/piece) and sugar-free mints (up to 2g/piece). As you can see, using diabetic products you can easily top 20g of sorbitol per meal. In one study with 39 healthy participants, 84% of them had symptoms of a sorbitol intolerance after consuming a 20g dose. Consumption of these products thus deserves caution.

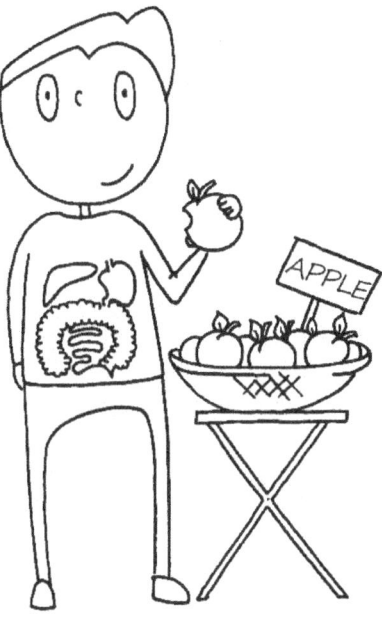

Man with sorbitol intolerance

Apples contain sorbitol by nature. On the picture, you see Tim, who does not know about his sorbitol intolerance. Due to it, he only has a limited amount of workers ensuring that the body makes use of the energy the sugar provides in his small intestine. By eating a whole apple, he puts them under a lot of pressure.

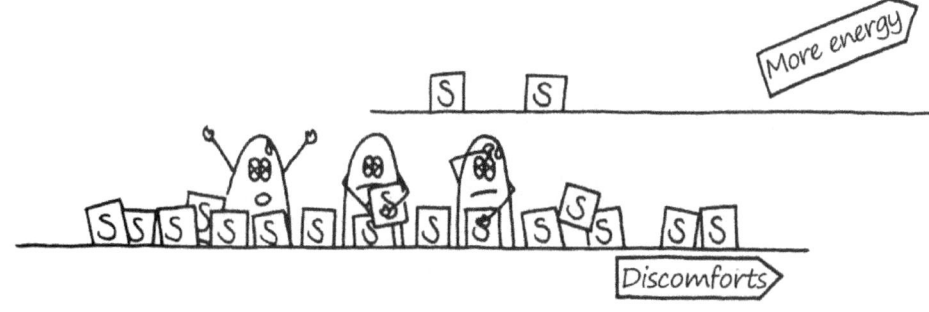

The load overstrains his workers. They are unable to handle the sudden amount of sorbitol and only put a fraction of them on the energy conveyor belt. The remainder arrives at the large intestine and thus causes symptoms.

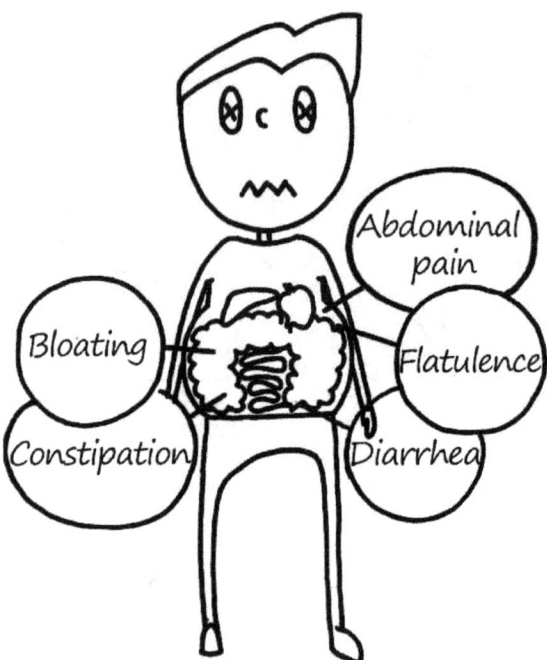

A few hours afterward the known assignation occurs—abdominal pain, bloating, diarrhea and flatulence.

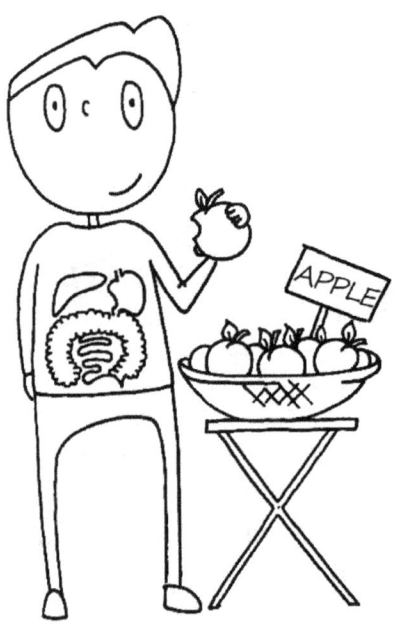

Man <u>without</u> sorbitol intolerance

With Chris, who is also eating an apple, it is entirely different.

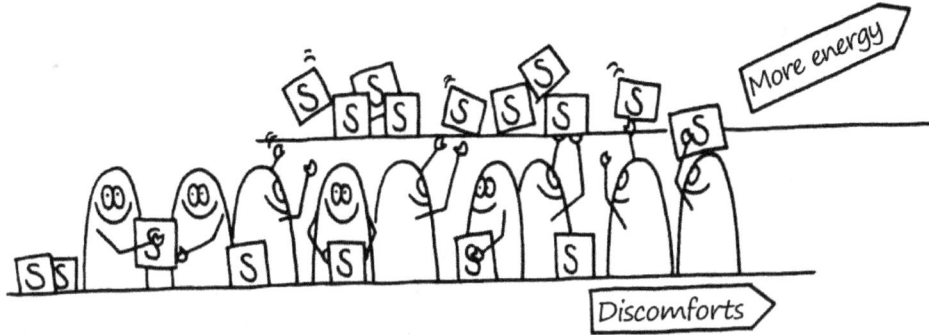

As he has no sorbitol intolerance and therefore many more workers, these can handle the sorbitol load with ease.

Your individual sensitivity

The task here is to limit your consumption of sorbitol-containing foods to the amount that your workers can cope with. The standard amount you find in the table is set to avoid sorbitol altogether. If you can tolerate some of it, though, you find the lower sensitivity level one amounts next to it. Reasons for the standard avoidance of sorbitol in case of an intolerance:

1. The breath test for sorbitol shows an intolerance present at 5g in **58%** of those experiencing abdominal discomfort due to an irritable bowel and **53%** of healthy participants (based on a combination of studies with 564 participants).
2. If you have a fructose intolerance, sorbitol will aggravate your symptoms. Sorbitol hinders the absorption of already-present fructose because fructose and sorbitol share a transportation mechanism where sorbitol is preferred.
3. Sugar-alcohols are causing symptoms to many and can sometimes even lead to a water aggregation in the small intestine, reducing the intestine's ability to metabolize nutrients. On average, 25–40% of consumed sugar-alcohols arrive at the colon. Even small amounts of sorbitol can trigger discomforts.

Hence, it makes sense to test whether you can tolerate more than the standard amounts in the tables in Chapter 3, as you want to be able to consume foods as deliberately as possible.

1.3.3 Consequences of a sorbitol intolerance

Physical effects

You are already familiar with the immediate effects of an untreated sorbitol intolerance: abdominal pain, bloating, diarrhea and flatulence. These alone are certainly enough to have you take action. However, indirectly they can also lead to lower lust, reduced social contacts, lower empathy and less vitality in general. Hence, not handling your intolerance lowers your quality of life. It is not so surprising that this also affects your days off work. A study, done in the USA and the Netherlands, shows that on average people with an untreated intolerance take about twice as many sick leaves from school or work than do their peers. Luckily, you can do something about that. You can recapture your well-being by learning how to adapt your diet to your capacity to absorb sorbitol. Ideally, you only limit your nutrition as far as is necessary—a certain amount of sorbitol may even be tolerable if you are intolerant towards sorbitol. My aim is to make this as easy as possible for you.

Depression

Note: The main studies underlying the following text included patients suffering from fructose and lactose intolerance only. Whether it also applies to fructans and galactans as well as sorbitol will be the topic of future examinations.

Scientists have found that there is a causal relation between having an untreated intolerance and increased depression scores. The reason for this is a reduced prevalence of a neurotransmitter, serotonin, in case fructose arrives at the large intestine. Serotonin elevates one's mood. The body produces it from tryptophan, which it derives from food. Presumably, at least, fructose that passes the small intestine—remains on the belt—merges with tryptophan to form a non-absorbable substance. This reaction reduces the amount of available tryptophan and causes the body to produce less serotonin. Hence, fructose that arrives at the large intestine hinders the body's ability to let positive feelings emerge. In an experiment in which patients lowered their fructose and sorbitol consumption, depression scores normalized for most participants. Keeping the consumption limits that apply to you when choosing your portion sizes can improve your mood (your serotonin metabolism) because fewer fructose arrives at the large intestine. Extra discipline is required to maintain the portion thresholds in cases of depression, however, as a lack of high spirits (tryptophan) can foster the hunger for sweets. Now, candies often contain fructose (and sorbitol).

If an intolerance is present, the intake of fructose containing sweets further lowers one's mood, creating a vicious circle.

You can find out how much you can eat for many foods in the lists in Chapter 3. Even if you are not depressed, please remember that in the presence of a dysfunctional metabolism, depression can result from consuming too much of foods that contain problematic ingredients. Affected people should always seek help rather than trying to counter these effects through sheer willpower and bear in mind that they can and should do something about ongoing feelings of sadness, little personal power, and low energy.

Summary

Bacteria ferment sorbitol—sugar-alcohols—if they reach the large intestine. In that case, they cause various abdominal symptoms. Many foods contain sorbitol. In case of a sorbitol intolerance, you have too few enzyme workers making sure your body uses sugar-alcohols to gain energy before it can reach the large intestine. You treat your symptoms by limiting your consumption of sorbitol to the capacity of your enzyme workers. To do so, you eat according to the tables in the third Chapter showing you the tolerated amount per meal. The lists enable you to savely reduce the amount of sorbitol as I used data for all nine sugar-alcohols to estimate your portion sizes (I am the first one that has done that). Moreover, you can enjoying as much freedom as is possible concerning your choice of foods, because I show you the tolerable amount in case of a low sorbitol sensitivity as well.

1.4 Background of an irritable bowel

Suffering from sorbitol intolerance symptoms is like having a sensitive colon. Like a notorious diva, your intestine shows a lack of robustness and an oversensitivity. It will not allow tampering with, reacts disappointed and offended when ignored by someone that offers her unfitting food. In the case of stress, she pipes up even more vehemently. Many people are carrying such a diva around with them, which repeatedly makes her demands known.

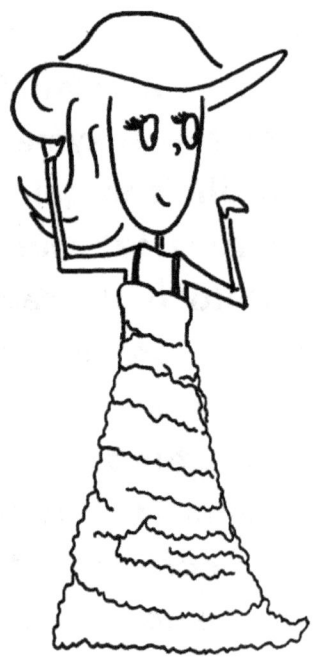

By the way, the exact causes of the diva's show up are unknown. In some cases, infections and emotions play a role. It seems like fortune decided who has a sorbitol intolerance and who does not. In any case, it has nothing to do with the character. Having a diva-tummy not at all means having a diva-like congeniality.

1.5 Abdominal discomfort in kids

In general, abdominal discomforts of your child can have a variety of reasons. A lactose intolerance will not occur before the age of five. Other potential triggers of abdominal pain, bloating and diarrhea in children are fructose and sorbitol: Children ages 14 to 58 months drank 250 mL of apple juice in a study. Afterward, all children who suffered from chronic diarrhea, as well as 65.5% of the healthy children, tested positive for malabsorption-symptoms. Avoiding apple juice led to recovery for **all** of the children. This result corresponds with other research that shows that many children suffer from diarrhea and abdominal pain if they drink too much fruit juice. Liquids that contain high levels of sorbitol are often the trigger. You should give your child a maximum of 10 mL juice per kilogram of body weight. Moreover, you should avoid giving them fruit juices that contain sorbitol or high amounts of free fructose, like apple or peach juice.

2

STRATEGY

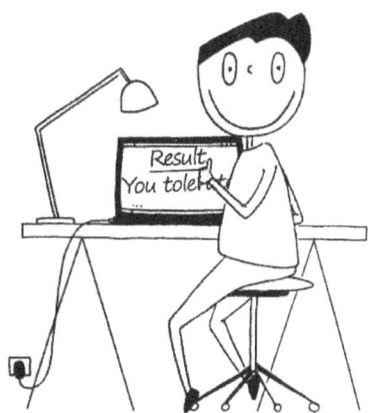

2.1   A gut's change management

No employee likes to stay at a company that always overstrains him. Equally unsatisfactory is to work at a place where one gets the feeling that one does not contribute at all. The typical consequences of both extremes: lack of motivation, an increase in the number of sick leaves up to an incapacity to work at the place anymore. What does that have to do with you? Quite simply: what goes in the professional environment, applies to your bowel as well. Hence, you should strive to work with your enzymes (conveyor-belt workers) in a team instead of over- or under-straining them. Show your leadership qualities and make your staff your motivated allies instead of waiting for them to come to you with their complaints!

How you can get that done, you will find out in this book. Did you ever want to rely on a master plan? If that is so, you will like what follows. According to the following plan, you will first determine the status quo of your symptoms. The next step is to keep a sorbitol diet for three weeks. At the end you determine, whether your symptoms have improved. If so, you can find out whether you can stomach more than the standard amounts—better adapt to the capacity of your workers. If your symptoms did not improve to your satisfaction, work on your stress level according to Chapter 2.8 or get *THE IBS NAVIGATOR* to search for alternative triggers.

2.1.1 Signpost

Status-quo-check: Note down your symptoms for four days **before** the diet

Introduction diet: Keep the the sorbitol diet according to the food tables in Chapter 3.

Efficiency check: Note down your symptoms on the last four days of your introductory diet to determine if the diet worked. If not, check alternative causes.

Adaption: Sensitivity check to find out if you can tolerate more than the standard serving sizes.

2.1.2 Roadmap

Step	Action	Target
Duty 1	**Status-quo-check** Fill out the symptom test sheet Duration: 4 days	Determining your status quo: Which symptoms do you have, and how severe are they?
Optional 2	**Breath tests at a specialist** Duration: 4 days	As you bought this book, you have either already taken it or done the substitute test in *THE IBS NAVIGATOR*. Otherwise, you can take the introductory diet to find out if the sorbitol diet works for you but it is more advisable to check for alternative triggers as well and for that, you need the book or a breath test.
Duty 3	**Introductory diet and efficiency check with symptom test sheet** Symptom tracking during the last four days of the diet. Duration of the diet: three weeks	You keep the sorbitol diet with the Chapter 3 tables and fill out the symptom test sheet. Did the diet lower your symptoms satisfactory? **Yes)** Continue with step four. **No)** Work on the stress management chapter. Another option is to check alternative triggers and diseases with *THE IBS NAVIGATOR*.
Optional 4	**Sensitivity-level-test** Duration: ~½ month	Enabling you a diet that is as varied as possible while reducing your symptoms is possible by determining your sensitivity level, see Chapter 4.

The goal of the overall strategy is to determine how much you tolerate without causing "the diva" to protest. The first step towards that goal it to determine the status quo, the severity of your symptoms, before changing your diet. The reason for this is that this is the only way to check, whether the diet has an effect. To do so, note down your discomforts in a copy of the following symptom test sheet. **Make sure to keep your symptom test sheets in a folder.** The days at which you note down your symptoms should be average to you. Neither a day on which you sickly vegetated in your bed nor one on which you celebrated the stag party of your best friend or had to master a difficult test count. If you are uncertain about whether it was an average day, cross it out. **Important: This also holds true for all of the subsequent tests. If you are in doubt as to whether the day was "normal," i.e. no circumstances distorted the symptoms, repeat the test to get a more reliable result.** On the days where you track your symptoms, always carry a copy of the symptom test sheet with you. Ideally, you should fill it out right after your main meals, e.g., at 7 am, 1 pm and 7 pm. After the four days of your status quo check, you should also be able to classify the type of stool you usually have. Depending on whether you have constipation, diarrhea or a mix of both, you are an IBS-C, IBS-D or IBS-M type. If you have neither constipation nor diarrhea, your IBS type is unclassified. Take that information with you when you visit the doctor. After tracking your symptoms for four days, follow the introductory diet. That means you keep a diet according to the tables in Chapter 3. In the last week, you then fill out the symptom test sheet to determine the diet's effectiveness. If keeping the diet leads to an improvement of your well-being that you are satisfied with, you should stick to it. You can read how to assess the test sheets more professionally than just laying the one before next to the one after the diet in Chapter 4.3. You can use the efficiency-check-symptom-sheet later as a reference for the sensitivity-level-test, if you decide to take it—it is also included in the advanced techniques-Chapter 4. With the latter, you can adjust to your enzyme worker's capacities to handle sorbitol.

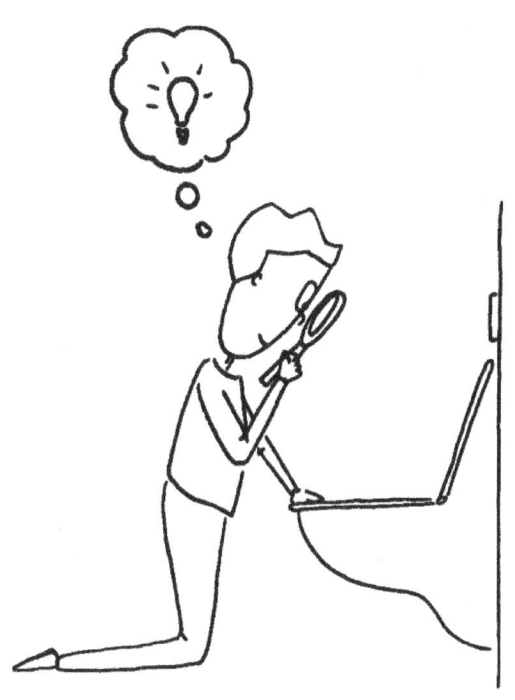

Stool types after Bristol

	Separate hard lumps, like nuts (hard to pass)	**Type** A: Constipation **Value** 4
	Sausage-shaped but lumpy	**Type** B: Constipation **Value** 2
	Like a sausage but with cracks on the surface	**Type** C: normal **Value** 1
	Like a sausage or snake, smooth and soft	**Type** D: normal **Value** 1
	Soft blobs with clear-cut edges	**Type** E: Diarrhoea **Value** 2
	Fluffy pieces with ragged edges, a mushy stool	**Type** F: Diarrhoea **Value** 4
	Watery, no solid pieces; **entirely liquid**	**Type** G: Diarrhoea **Value** 5

(Based on Lewis & Heaton, 1997; Thompson, 2006)

Types 3 and 4 are the norm. The farther away your type is from these two, the worse your ailments.

2.1.3 Symptom test sheet

Note down your stool type in the morning 🐓, afternoon ☀, and evening ☾ and your stool value from 1 to 5 (see page 24) as well as the number of times you visited the toilet to estimate the stool grade by multiplying the numbers. Also, evaluate bloating and pain from 1 to 5 according to the following scale:

1. No discomfort, like someone without symptoms
2. Hardly any discomfort relative to someone without symptoms
3. Medium discomfort relative to someone without symptoms
4. Severe discomfort relative to someone without symptoms
5. Very severe discomfort relative to someone without symptoms

Test:_____ **End date:**_____

For each test, you need copies of this page!

		Type/ Value	Defecation count		Stool grade	+	Bloating grade	+	Pain grade	= B
Day 1 prior	🐓		x		=					**TEST DAY**
	☀		x		=(+)	+		+		
	☾		x		=(+)	+		+		
		The day's sum	A =		=		=			
Day 2 prior	🐓		x		=					**Day 1 after**
	☀		x		=(+)	+		+		
	☾		x		=(+)	+		+		
		The day's sum	A =		=		=			
Day 3 prior	🐓		x		=					**Day 2 after**
	☀		x		=(+)	+		+		
	☾		x		=(+)	+		+		
		The day's sum	A =		=		=			
Day 4 prior)	🐓		x		=					**Day 3 after**
	☀		x		=(+)	+		+		
	☾		x		=(+)	+		+		
		The day's sum	A =		=		=			

LAXIBA®

Example: The four status quo (1.)/Level (2.) check days

Note down your stool type in the morning 🐓, afternoon ☀, and evening ☾ and your stool value from 1 to 5 (see page 24) as well as the number of times you visited the toilet to estimate the stool grade by multiplying the numbers. Also, evaluate bloating and pain from 1 to 5 according to the following scale:

1. No discomfort, like someone without symptoms
2. Hardly any discomfort relative to someone without symptoms
3. Medium discomfort relative to someone without symptoms
4. Severe discomfort relative to someone without symptoms
5. Very severe discomfort relative to someone without symptoms

Test:_____ **End date:**_____

For each test, you need copies of this page!

		Type/Value	Defecation count		Stool grade	Bloating grade	Pain grade	
Day 1 prior	🐓	E 2	x 2	=	4	2	2	**TEST DAY**
	☀	F 4	x 2	=(+)	8	+ 2	+ 3	
	☾	E 2	x 2	=(+)	4	+ 3	+ 2	
		The day's sum		=	16	= 7	= 7	
Day 2 prior	🐓	F 4	x 2	=	8	2	3	**Day 1 after**
	☀	E 2	x 1	=(+)	2	+ 3	+ 4	
	☾	F 4	x 1	=(+)	4	+ 2	+ 2	
		The day's sum		=	14	= 7	= 9	
Day 3 prior	🐓	E 2	x 1	=	2	2	3	**Day 2 after**
	☀	F 4	x 2	=(+)	8	+ 2	+ 4	
	☾	E 2	x 1	=(+)	2	+ 3	+ 5	
		The day's sum		=	12	= 7	= 12	
Day 4 prior)	🐓	F 4	x 1	=	4	2	2	**Day 3 after**
	☀	E 2	x 1	=(+)	2	+ 2	+ 2	
	☾	F 4	x 2	=(+)	8	+ 3	+ 3	
		The day's sum		=	14	= 7	= 7	

LAXIBA® THE SORBITOL NAVIGATOR

Example: The four efficiency check days

Note down your stool type in the morning 🐓, afternoon ☀, and evening ☾ and your stool value from 1 to 5 (see page 24) as well as the number of times you visited the toilet to estimate the stool grade by multiplying the numbers. Also, evaluate bloating and pain from 1 to 5 according to the following scale:

1. No discomfort, like someone without symptoms
2. Hardly any discomfort relative to someone without symptoms
3. Medium discomfort relative to someone without symptoms
4. Severe discomfort relative to someone without symptoms
5. Very severe discomfort relative to someone without symptoms

Test:_____ **End date:**_____

For each test, you need copies of this page!

		Type/ Value	Defecation count		Stool grade	Bloating grade	Pain grade	
Day 1 prior	🐓	-	x 0	=	0	1	1	**TEST DAY**
	☀	E 2	x 1	=(+)	2	+ 1	+ 1	
	☾	D 1	x 1	=(+)	1	+ 1	+ 1	
			The day's sum	=	3	= 3	= 3	
Day 2 prior	🐓	D 1	x 1	=	1	1	1	**Day 1 after**
	☀	-	x 0	=(+)	0	+ 1	+ 1	
	☾	D 1	x 1	=(+)	1	+ 1	+ 1	
			The day's sum	=	2	= 3	= 3	
Day 3 prior	🐓	D 1	x 1	=	1	1	1	**Day 2 after**
	☀	-	x 0	=(+)	0	+ 2	+ 2	
	☾	E 2	x 1	=(+)	2	+ 1	+ 1	
			The day's sum	=	3	= 4	= 4	
Day 4 prior)	🐓	-	x 0	=	0	1	1	**Day 3 after**
	☀	D 1	x 1	=(+)	1	+ 1	+ 1	
	☾	D 1	x 1	=(+)	1	+ 1	+ 1	
			The day's sum	=	2	= 3	= 3	

2.1.4 Keeping your balance

Now, you know if the diet provides you benefits and maybe even, how sensitive you are. Still, aside from avoiding the consumption of too much of your trigger, you should also learn some generally advisable nutrition principles.

1	Eat a rich variety of foods, i.e., something different each day and with lots of natural ingredients. Eat with a relaxed posture.	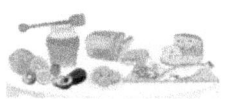
2	Take care of your supply of fiber, e.g., by eating potatoes, flax seeds, lentils, nuts.	
3	Ingest five portions of vegetables (ideally dark green, red or orange) and fruit.	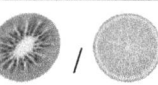 5/day
4	Have some reduced-fat milk products like reduced-fat milk, yogurt or cheese every day.	
5	One or two times a week, eat fish and eggs, as well as 300–600g of low-fat meat, ideally poultry.	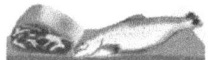
6	Use vegetable oils if possible, like canola oil, and fats.	
7	Reduce your consumption of salt and sugar.	
8	Drink at least 1.5 liters of non-alcoholic drinks per day. Best are unsweetened beverages and water. Drink alcohol moderately or avoid it entirely.	
9	Preferably, cook fresh and at lower temperatures to reduce nutrient leaching.	
+	Stay fit: exercise regularly.	

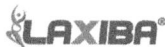

Summary

As part of the strategy, you first note down your symptoms before doing anything. Then you start the introductory diet. For it, you reduce the consumption of sorbitol containing foods. The aim is to check whether the diet lowers your symptoms after all. So, fill out the symptom-test-sheet before starting the diet. Then follow the diet according to the tables in Chapter 3 for three weeks and fill out the test-sheet once more for the last four days. If you are feeling better now, you can also determine your precise sensitivity level; see Chapter 4. If you still have symptoms, follow steps two and three as described on the next page.

Make sure you keep a balanced diet:
Drink least 1.5 liters of water per day and exercise regularly. Also, ensure to eat a variety of foods, to supply your body with the vitamins that are important for your health. To achieve that, regularly eat fruits and vegetables.

2.2 Your individual strategy

This Chapter describes how to proceed accurately with the introduction of diet and the sensitivity level test. During the introductory diet, you keep the portions stated in the tables in Chapter 3. Please note here that the tolerated portions refer to one meal—expecting three meals at intervals of about six hours per day. Follow these steps:

First, you take the introductory diet according to the sorbitol standard amounts in the food tables in Chapter 3. Four days before starting the diet as well as on the last four days of the third week, you fill out the symptom test sheet on page 25. With it, you can determine the diet's success see Chapter 4.3. The diet is efficient; however, if after three weeks of keeping it, you should not find any improvement, find out whether you unwillingly consumed too much sorbitol. One way to do so is to keep a nutrition diary and check it with a specialist or nutrition consultant. If you ruled out an accidental intake of sorbitol, and are unhappy with the improvement of your well-being, improve your stress management according to Chapter 2.8. Aside from that, you can use *THE IBS NAVIGATOR* to test for a fructans and galactans sensitivity and perform alternative strategies.

The test procedure in three levels of escalation

Subsequently, you find an example of the test process for someone with sorbitol intolerance:

1) Reduce your sorbitol consumption according to the sorbitol tables in Chapter 3 for three weeks. Fill out the symptom test sheet for four days before the diet as well as on the last four days. In the third week, if your discomforts improved satisfactory, keep the sorbitol diet. If you like, you can adjust your sensitivity level further (see Chapter 4). If you remain dissatisfied, act according to step 2).
2) Improve your stress management according to Chapter 2.8.
3) Get *THE IBS NAVIGATOR* and repeat the introduction with fructans and galactans as well. Did your symptoms improve further? If so, keep this diet. In case you are still searching for an improvement, check the alternative strategies chapter in that book.

2.2.1 Substitute test

You want to check, whether you can stomach fructose but your expert is unable to offer you a breath test? For this case, I have developed the substitute test. As you determine the result based on your symptoms, it is necessary to rule out the influence of alternative triggers. Thus, you need *THE IBS NAVIGATOR* to do the test. In it, you will find the extensive explanation and the instruction to perform the substitute test.

2.2.2 It depends on the total load

You feel discomfort as soon as too much sorbitol arrives at your small intestine for your enzyme workers to handle. The more sorbitol, the worse your symptoms are. In the food tables in the third Chapter of the book, you will find the portion sizes that fit your sensitivity. What do you do if you want to combine different foods, e.g., as you prepare to cook a recipe, if you tolerate a limited amount of some of them? If you used the maximum amount of sorbitol for the cucumber already, do you have to deny yourself the tomatoes? Nonessential: reduce the consumption for one or several of the sorbitol containing foods far enough to not surpass the amount thresholds in sum. Makes sense? Not yet? Here is another example: your sensitivity for sorbitol is low (in the food tables, you use the second column for your diet) and would like to prepare a fruit yogurt for breakfast. For it, you intend to mix mango (of which you can tolerate 4 tablespoons with 15g each) and nectarine (of it you can tolerate one tablespoon with 15g). Hence, both foods contain sorbitol. In order avoid surpassing your tolerance threshold; restrict yourself to two tablespoons of magno and half a tablespoon of nectarine. Thus, the total amount of sorbitol you consume at the meal is below your threshold. If the reduced amounts are too small for you, you may want to look for alternatives. In Chapter 3.7.1, you can find various fruits. Oranges for example are sorbitol free.

2.3 Prevalence of the intolerances

According to an extensive current study in Switzerland, 27% of people with abdominal discomfort suffer from a fructose intolerance, 17% from a lactose intolerance and a further 33% from both. However, the fructose dose of 35g that the study used is high for European conditions, if a Finnish study from 1987 still applies to contemporary diets, and low for American conditions, wherein the average daily amount consumed is 54g. Hence, there is no fixed reference around the world. Another research study using 25g fructose as its base level suggests only a 49% average prevalence of fructose intolerance. An analysis of several studies shows that independent from the investigations mentioned above, 58% of those with irritable bowel symptoms have a sorbitol intolerance. There are no research results concerning the prevalence of a fructans and galactans intolerance known to me at this point.

Are you surprised about the low level of lactose intolerance? Well, you have to account for the fact that it is lowest for Caucasians as they adapted to tolerate milk to cope better with less sunshine in a day. Still, I was amazed that lactose intolerance is not the common type of intolerances according to the studies I read. If you stroll through supermarkets, however, you will hardly find a shelf that holds products for people with sorbitol or fructose intolerance. Instead, the markets have adjusted solely on lactose intolerance—also concerning the labeling. Those suffering from sorbitol intolerance have to learn the names of nine sugar-alcohols and their assignment numbers instead. Go to page 48, to find out more.

2.4 General diet hints

2.4.1 Good reasons for your persistence

Imagine that one of your best friends goes on a two-week vacation leaving his beloved Labrador retriever, *Bailey*, in your care, along with some instructions about the dog's health needs as it has an intolerance towards an ingredient in some dog foods. You run out of dog food after the first week, just as you sat down on the couch to relax—not planning to leave the house again for today. Now you remember that you still have a can of the food you give to the square like dog of your auntie in the basement. If you give *Bailey* some of that, you save an hour drive to the store and back as well as going outside where it started to rain. Annoyingly, the food for your aunt's dog contains the trigger *Bailey* has to avoid. Unlike the happy dog image on the package suggests, giving him this food causes him pain, flatulence, and lethargy; catching a stick will be out of the question for this poor pooch. Maybe, you also imagine your aunt, whose dog feels well even after consuming what you would never feed him—you remember a cream pie that fell victim to that bitch. "Hogwash!" she would say. "Dogs can eat anything! A dog intolerance—if he only eats enough there will be no farts!"

What is your position at that moment? Back on the couch or driving through the rain to the expert dealer? Now, I am relieved. Therefore, the dog of your friend is worth spending time and money as well as acting considerably. If, at any point it becomes difficult for you to keep your diet, think about the happy *Bailey* and send the square couch potato dog back to your aunt's home!

In the end, I call upon you to take responsibility for your nutrition. Show respect to your body. Acquire the necessary courage and discipline. Your body is a part of you. Just as many vegetarians stand by their dietary choices for the duration of their lives, you should stand by your diet and your body. Be yourself. The key is not starting out perfect but starting at all and making small improvements every day. That is something you can do! You have the courage and *Bailey* will give you the courage.

Your target should be to change your sustenance day by day, food by food, in such a way as to allow you to lead a mostly symptom-free life. All beginnings are difficult, however, and as you leap the initial hurdles, you will find further motivation and discipline in discovering how much your nutritional changes are paying off for you.

The first step in that direction is to connect that goal with whatever is most important to you in your life. Independent of where your passions lie, you will enjoy them better by gaining more energy and improved wellbeing.

Do you not believe me? Then imagine *Bailey* once more: The retriever sneaks through the house and as he sees a cat pass by through the window, his only reaction is to fart. Then, he retreats into his dog hatchet with an abdominal cramp, curing the food for the aunt's dog that got him into the hot water. You do not want to end up likewise. What about this instead: The retriever sneaks through the house, hears steps, stalks to the open window, stops and sees what looks like a burglar nearby the post box (he does not see the letters in his hands). In a flash, *Bailey* is on the road right behind him giving him a good bark! Pure energy!

What is your passion? What is your affair of the heart? Gain strength by keeping a diet that is best for you and give it a fresh start. Turn your attention and abilities toward eating in a way that will help you achieve your goals. If you are uncertain whether you can reach, your goals do this: Imagining that you have already done it. How? Cut out the following card and fold it as indicated. Then put it somewhere you can see it every day. Ideally, you can take a picture of yourself after a particularly fruitful milestone and put it on the drawing. Then let it encourage you to continue improving your nutrition each day. *Stephen William Hawking* has never stopped producing outstanding scientific works despite suffering from a myasthenia. Why? Because he is following his heart and because he has a positive attitude about life. Who seeks excuses when they are passionate about something? When it comes to passion, it is all about the how. It is about doing what is possible and thus it is always all about the solution. There are similar examples in sports. *Melissa Stockwell* achieves first class athletic performance despite having lost a leg. Her sport is her passion, and she finds ways to excel in it regardless of the circumstances life gave her.

So what is your passion? Write it down. Then make it clear to yourself that a symptom-reducing diet will positively affect your achievement. Then get on your way to making this nutrition a part of your life. In addition—always remember about your friend, *Bailey*, the dog.

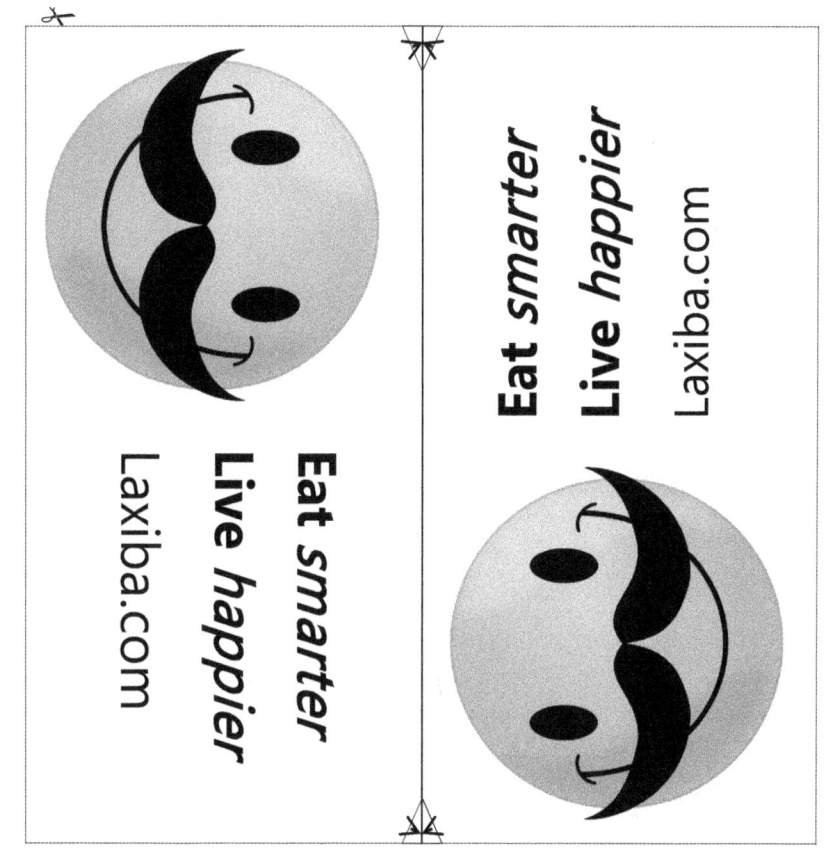

2.4.2 Mealtimes

Even when and how often you eat can affect your digestion. Who better to ask on that subject than athletes? They, in particular, depend on an optimal nutrient supply. The analysis shows that over 97% of elite Canadian athletes eat at least three times a day; 57% of them also take a snack in the morning, 71% in the afternoon and 58% in the evening. Moreover, regular mealtimes have a positive effect on the cardiovascular system. A study of more than 4,500 children showed that the risk of childhood obesity markedly decreases the more often children eat during the day. How is that? Well, ask the mail carrier of *Bailey's* owner, whether he dares bringing him his letters after eating a gravitationally detrimental meal, his daily ration, in the morning.

2.4.3 Eating out

At home, restricting one's consumption of trigger containing foods is rather easy. Now you want to eat at a restaurant of a friend's house so what do you do? Of course, you understand that a restaurant staff usually does not have the dietician's expertise required to tell you the ingredients of each meal. Luckily, you can help yourself. For example by learning about some foods that you can usually eat without having to think about them. These include eggs, fish or meat without breading or sauce, kiwis, leafy salads dressed with oil, oregano, pepper and salt, oranges, basil pesto, potatoes, rice, and tortillas. You have to be careful with diabetic products and prepared sauces, as they often contain sorbitol. What about menus, however? Have you ever spent time at a restaurant considering what the ideal combination of menu items would be for you? The good thing is that you can often ask for a change to menu items without paying extra if you ask the server. You can likewise voice your needs to your hosts when you receive an invitation to a meal. To make it easy, just hand out the safe products list (see Chapter 2.6). You can send it out with the following message, for example:

"Dear [name of the host],

I was glad to receive your invitation to [occasion like your wedding], and I am happy to come. If it is possible for you to cook some of the foods that are included in the attached table separately from the other meals, then I can take part in the meal, as well. Please tell me whether that will be possible so that I can plan accordingly.

Thank you and see you soon!

[Your name]"

The safe products list, see Chapter 2.6, also makes it easier for a restaurant kitchen to find a suitable meal for you. As fast food chains are not as readily equipped to adapt their menus, you will find many fast food chain products and the portion sizes you can stomach in the third part of this book. You can stay on the safe side by always having your book with you. However, it will hardly be always at hand, unlike a foldable list for your purse or wallet. In Chapter 2.5 you will find the cheat sheet with the tolerable portion sizes of some common products. This list also includes information on sorbitol names.

2.4.4 Convenience foods

Unfortunately, sorbitol is a part of many convenience foods or is naturally contained in the ingredients. However, you will find exceptions, even when shopping on the cheap, including convenience foods that advertise the use of natural ingredients and those that contain basil pesto. The cheat sheet (see Chapter 2.5) will inform you of which ingredients on a package mean that the food contains sorbitol.

2.4.5 Medicine and oral hygiene

Anything you take into your mouth can cause symptoms if it contains sorbitol. In particular, it is included in many oral hygiene products. An example of a sorbitol-free toothpaste is *JASON® healthy mouth*. Moreover, use dental floss without wax, and find a mouthwash such as *TheraBreath® Fresh Breath Oral Rinse*. It sometimes gets tricky, as sorbitol is not always obvious as an ingredient. If you are in doubt, call the customer service hotline of the respective product and ask them for clarification.

The search for sorbitol-free medicines may be especially hard, so ask your pharmacist for assistance. Many nasal sprays, eye drops, and expectorants contain this additive. However, if you look hard enough, you will usually find alternatives for these as well. Examples of sorbitol-free pharmaceuticals include: *Allegra® 12 Hour Allergy* (allergy), *Allerest® PE Allergy & Sinus Relief—Tablets* (frontal sinusitis), *Ayr® Saline Nasal Rinse Kit* (frontal sinusitis), *Florax® DS Diarrhea Relief Vials* (diarrhea), *Hyland's® Earache—Drops* (earache), *Mucinex® 12 Hour Extended Release Expectorant—Tablets* (expectorant), *Mucinex® Sinus-Max Severe Congestion Relief—Tablets* (frontal sinusitis), *SinuCleanse® Neti Pot All Natural Nasal Wash System* (frontal sinusitis) and *Visine-A® Eye Allergy Relief, Antihistamine & Redness Reliever, Drops* (allergy).

Despite your best efforts at researching your intolerance, you may find yourself unable to stomach medicine for whatever reason. If you are having symptoms, search for alternatives. If in doubt, use the symptom-test-sheet. Write down your symptoms while using it and compare it with a record of your diet taken when you were not using the medicine, for example, on your efficiency check sheet. You can use any sheet where you recorded your symptoms after refraining from sorbitol.

2.4.6 Nutritional supplements

If you take vitamin supplements, the following examples are sorbitol-free:

Nature's Bounty® Vitamin B-12, 1000mcg, *Nature Made® Vitamin B6 100mg Dietary Supplement Tablets*, *Walgreens® Multivitamin Ultimate Men's Tablets*, *Walgreens® Multivitamin Ultimate Women's Tablets*. A long-term trial did not prove the use of multivitamin supplements. If you take them, make sure not to take too much of certain vitamins. Vitamins that can be unsafe in excess include *B3, B6,* as well as *A, D, E* and *K*, which can cause symptoms of poisoning if you overdose. Thus, you should discuss your intake with your doctor. A viable approach with these vitamins is taking them in three-month cycles. That means taking them for three months and then taking the next three months off.

2.4.7 Protein shakes—nutrition for athletes

There is a partially questionable trend among athletes to take special supplements. If you can cover your protein demand with the products listed in Chapter 2.1.4, you have no need for protein shakes or the like. Some energy bars and electrolyte products contain sorbitol (see Chapter 3.2). You can often find trigger free alternatives in pharmacies.

2.4.8   Fish and meat

Fish and meat by nature are free of sorbitol. Nevertheless, you have to be careful with sauce, which may contain sorbitol. To find out that, check the list of ingredients of the product.

2.4.9   These actions lead to lasting change

To achieve lasting success, it is important that you monitor your nutrition. If you find yourself starting to ignore the recommended amounts, you should get back on track and restart your commitment as soon as possible. Write down your goal to adapt your nutrition to the stated food and drink portion sizes to reduce abdominal discomfort and improve your quality of life. Stay conscious of the negative consequences of eating "blindly" covered in the first part of this book. Why is it important to change your habits? Re-read your goal and then write down your five most important reasons for striving toward it. Moreover, answer the following question. Why it is important to act **now**?

Probably, you have made the following experience as well. Filled with motivation and enthusiasm you plunge into something, like a New Year's resolution. One goes right after it and even celebrates first successes. However, this feeling trickles away unless soon afterward even bigger successes surpass the first one. If that does not happen, a slight inertia arises. If you change your diet, this can happen to you as well. It is like there is an angel on your one shoulder to whom you say that you are going to keep at it even if it becomes arduous yet there is an imp sitting on your other shoulder, which is already laughing at his sleeve. In fact, the way gets steeper after the first yards. Many then let things slide, which makes further successes impossible, and the symptoms come back. "Isn't that unfair?" the imp is telling you, "you are putting in your effort for days and how does it pay off? You are having the same symptoms as you had before. Let it be." The angel may have screamed so much that it is croaky by now and shrugs his shoulders exhaustedly. "Sorry, but I tried my best," one excuses oneself trying not to look at the grinning devil.

It is a cognitive bias to believe that it is easier just to accept one's symptoms than to change your diet to avoid them. What about you? Did you catch yourself close to giving up? If so, send the devil on your shoulder to the desert where it belongs.

I can promise you: After you changed your diet to fit your food's sorbitol content, you will have more energy and a higher quality of life. In addition, after you have mastered staying on the right path for some month, you will find that you are getting used to it, which will make it even easier to stick with it. Getting used to it is something that the imp has deliberately concealed: Once you have taken the first pitch, you get accustomed to quickly assessing foods about their content of sorbitol and learns to notice sorbitol hideouts. Juggling with the amounts becomes so easy that you do not have to think long. At the start, the cheat sheet and this book will serve you well. Later you no longer need both as you know yourself what is right for you. The imp that you sent to the desert now is hot with anger, and you are the one that has a big grin on the face. You have the best arguments to be tenacious!

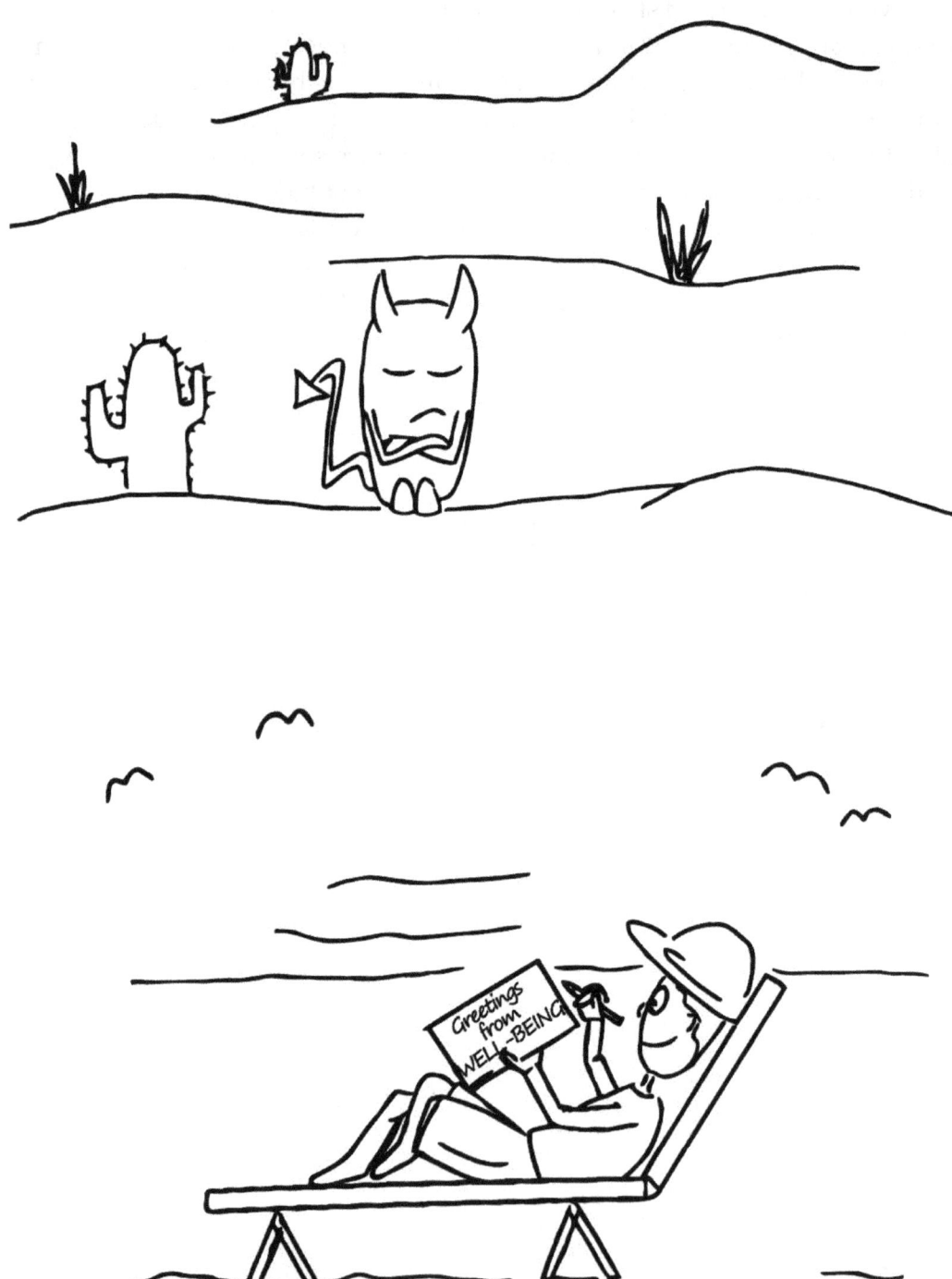

Are you uncertain as to whether you are going to remain motivated? Create an objective agreement with yourself. Note down in writing, why it pays off to you, to endure. Which goal do you want to achieve? For example, like this:

Objective agreement (write it down yourself)

What: comply with the acceptable amounts – Send the devil to the desert.

How to measure it: daily at 7:45 pm (set an alarm on your phone): did I comply with the portion restrictions?

Consequence: YES, you complied, so give yourself a small reward. NO, you did not so do 10 pushups or mow the lawn (anything you can do, which is good for you but you do not like doing).

Get it done: start within three days and keep on actively managing your diet until you have formed a habit of doing it.

Activities: Put this book into your kitchen and the cheat sheet into your wallet; inform those close to you; create reminders in your flat and your car, place your objective agreement somewhere where you can see it at least once a day (e.g. your mirror).

A good way to ensure that you stay committed is to integrate your spouse. Ask them to motivate you and to reflect back to you, which positive changes they notice about you. Another option is to book one of our coaches at *https://laxiba.com/trainer* to help you implement the steps explained in this book. What is more, you will find a way to talk with others and motivate each other at *https://laxiba.com/team*.

The more vivid and multifaceted you can imagine your life after a successful conversion of your diet, the more likely you are to keep moving forward with it and doing what is necessary. Have you been in a rut one day? Forget about it; get the job done better the day after! You can use this book as a compass and correct your course back to being well!

2.4.10 Reasons for using sorbitol

Why for example is sorbitol included in some soft drinks and sweets? Sorbitol makes products free from table sugar to enable diabetics to consume them as well as keeps chocolates moist. For drugs, sorbitol is a carrier for active substances because it is simple and works well. There would be alternatives that work well in many cases, which would not cost much more. So far, there is no strong lobby against using sorbitol in foods or making them easier to avoid, yet. Of course, sorbitol also occurs naturally, but that is not a valid reason to use it instead of the also naturally occurring Stevia in, for example, chewing gums.

2.4.11 Positive aspects of the diet

Do you want to disagree with me after reading the headline? For many the sorbitol diet equals abdication. In its original sense, however, diet (from the Greek díaita) means "lifestyle" or "way of life." Are abdication and the feeling of a downer an accurate description of the lifestyle that you want? On the contrary, you perform the diet to lower you symptoms and thus increases your quality of life. As you find out, which foods you can eat concerning the sorbitol content, you will automatically start thinking about what you eat in general. The chances are that you will end up eating healthier, and healthy is a much friendlier summary of your lifestyle. Of course, an alternative to the diet would be the use of medicine, like painkillers or drugs to stop diarrhea. Better yet, is to make sure symptoms do not occur in first place.

2.4.12 Testing yourself

Some of those affected struggle to absorb other ingredients like aspartame or maltodextrin. If you have reason to believe that this applies to you, follow the alternative introductory diet outlined in *THE IBS NAVIGATOR*.

2.4.13 Sweetener's sorbitol content

Pure stevia is sorbitol-free. Aside from that, sorbitol is contained in many sweeteners as well as light and sugar-free products.

Summary

A healthy, balanced diet, fixed mealtimes, and regular exercise are important not only in case of a sorbitol intolerance but for all people. Unfortunately, sometimes sorbitol is included in products although sorbitol free alternatives are available. Hence, especially when eating convenience foods or taking drugs, watch out for sorbitol in the ingredients. Stick to the sorbitol diet if it works. The longer you persist, the easier it gets to maintain it.

2.5 The cheat sheet

Cut out the leaflet on the following page. Please fold it along the thick lines. Start with the dotted line. Then fold it again at the half-dashed line. You can now keep this important information at hand when you are out and about or shopping.

Flyer sorbitol intolerance

Tolerated in case of sorbitol intolerance are

Maltodextrin	Sorbic acid	Barley malt syrup
Sodium sorbate	Potassium sorbate	Calcium sorbate
Sorbitan...	Polyoxyethylene(20)-sorbitan...	

(INS add. numbers: 200-203, 432-436, 491-495)

These ingredients are sugar alcohols:

Sorbitol	Mannitol	Xylitol	Hexanhexol
Lactitol	(Ethyl-) Maltol	Inositol	
Glucitol	Maltitol/-syrup	Sionon	
Isomalt	Palatinit®		
Erythritol	Pinitol		

(INS add. numbers: 420-21, 636-37, 953, 965-7)

Hence, avoid foods that contain them.

Only copy with permission. Copyright © 2016 Jan Stratbucker

Sugar alcohols like sorbitol are often contained in:

- Diabetics and dietary products
- Athletes products and energy bars
- Convenience foods and sauces
- Chewing gum and mints except for those that only contain stevia and table sugar
- Some light and isotonic beverages
- Drugs and mouthwashes
- Bars, chocolates, cream, and cream pies
- Moreover, some fruits, their juices, and alcoholic beverages as well as some vegetables

Interior left

Sorbitol intolerance portion sizes

Pineapple ¾ P-140g
Apple ☹² E; 182g
Apricots ¾ E; 35g
Vinegar balsa. 23 P-15g
Banana 9¼ E; 118g
Blueberry Muffin 88 E; 113g
Beer 10 G-200ml
Big Mac® 6½ E; 215g
Bitter Lemon ☺
Pear ¼ E; 15g
Lettuces 3 P-85g
Cauliflower 2½ P-85g

Broccoli ☺
Blackberries ☹² P-140g
Cranberries 45¼ P-55g
Froot Loops® ☺
Coca Cola® ☺
Corn Flakes ☺ P-30g
Strawberries ¼ P-140g
Special K® original ☺
Garden salad 16 P-85g
Ginger Ale ☺
Cucumber 1 E; 85g
Oats ☺

If you are sensitive avoid any food but one with ☺

Portion unit abbreviations (gram follows):

Exemplar	Cup	Glas	Portion	Tbsp.
E	C	G	P	T

☹=avoid; ☺=nearly free; ☺=is free of it

Only copy with permission. Copyright © 2016 Jan Stratbucker

Interior right

Chicken sweet and sour ☺
Raspberries 1½ P-140g
Honey 1¾ T; 15g
Currants 2½ P-140g
Coffee ☺
Potatoes 45¼ P-110g
Ketchup 3¾ T; 15g
Cherries ¼ T; 15g
Kiwi ☺
Cabbage 58¾ P-85g
Pumpkin butternut ☺
Long Island Icet. 16 G-200ml
M & M's® ☺
Mango 4 T; 15g
Mate tea ☺
Mayonnaise ☺
Melon 14¼ P-140g
Milk ☺
Granola bar ☹²
Nectarines 1 T; 15g
Oranges ☺ E; 140g

Peppers ☺ E; 85g
Pepsi® ☺ G-200ml
Peach ¼ E; 140g
Plum ¾ T; 15g
Mushroom ¾ T; 15g
Pizza ¾ E; 209g
Red Bull® ☺
Rice ☺
Sauerkraut ¾ T; 15g
Chocolate 48 P-25g
Champaign ¾ G-200ml
Smacks® 83¼ P-30g
Sushi 1½ P-140g
Tomatoes 1 T; 85g
Grapes ½ P-140g
Wine ¾ G-200ml
Wheat bread 26¼ P-42g
Whopper® 1 E; 315g
Lemon ☺
Chewing gum light ☺
7UP® ☺

LAXIBA

Cheat sheet content

To determine sorbitol-free products, you, unfortunately, have to navigate an unbelievable minefield of identifiers, despite the high prevalence of the condition:[1]

Caution, these foods often contain sugar-alcohols like sorbitol:

- Diabetic and dietary products
- Electrolyte products and energy bars
- Convenience foods and prepared sauces
- Chewing gums and mints, except those sweetened only with Stevia, for example. Sorbitol is either only contained in traces or not contained at all in Wrigley's® Spearmint, Doublemint and Juicy Fruit
- Some "light," i.e., sugar-free, and isotonic beverages
- Medicine and oral hygiene products
- Bars, pralines, sweet pastries, tarts, prepared cream
- Puréed, pickled or breaded sausages, fish, and meat

Moreover, some fruits (like apples, apricots, bananas, cantaloupe, carambola, cherries, cranberries, grapes, guava, lowbush cranberries, mango, nectarine, peach, pear, pineapple, plum, pomegranate, raspberries, strawberries and watermelon) and vegetables (artichoke, asparagus, beets, cabbage, carrots, cauliflower, celeriac, celery, chestnuts, chicory, coleslaw, cucumber, eggplant, endive, fennel bulb, garbanzo beans (chickpeas), kale, kohlrabi, leeks, lettuce (Boston), lettuce (green leaf), lettuce (iceberg), lettuce (red leaf), lettuce (romaine), mushrooms, olives, onions, pickled beets, radish, sauerkraut, sour pickles, soybean sprouts, spinach, tempeh, tomatoes and turnip), including juices contain sorbitol. Many alcoholic beverages do, as well, but brandy, gin, rum and whiskey, for example, are often sorbitol-free.

---

[1] There is an immediate need for simplification here. A proper solution is the declaration "contains sorbitol".

Noncritical ingredients for sorbitol intolerance[2]

Maltodextrin	Sorbic acid	Barley malt syrup
Sodium sorbate	Potassium sorbate	Calcium sorbate
Sorbitan...	Polyoxyethylene (20) –sorbitan-...	

Critical ingredients for sorbitol intolerance[3]

Sorbitol	Mannitol	Xylitol
Lactitol	(Ethyl-) Maltol	Hexanhexol
Glucitol	Maltitol/-syrup	Inositol
Isomalt	Palatinit®	Sionon
Erythritol	Pinitol	

---

[2] INS additive numbers: 200–203, 432–436, 491–495.
[3] INS additive numbers: 420–21, 636–37, 953, 965–67.

2.6 The safe products list

Likely, if you yourself do not have a sorbitol intolerance, someone in your circle of acquaintances has the irritable bowel syndrome or an intolerance towards some ingredient. As a good host, you may have already been in a situation to consider those to make sure that none of your guests encounters an uneasy feeling after an invitation.

If you ask your guests to tell you about any problematic ingredient you should accustom to, you are prepared professionally: Such a question will always leave a positive impression as it shows that your guest's well-being is important to you. You are well accustomed to any guest, if you make sure that some foods that are usually tolerable for anyone are on the menu. How can you achieve that? It is quite simple: make sure to offer the sauces separately from the side dishes. Hence, provide a bowl of potatoes, another bowl with butter, a third one with salad and lastly one with dressings. By the way, with some exceptions like garlic and onions anyone can tolerate most herbs and spices. The table on the following page shows you some usually safe foods.

Fruit	Vegetables	Warm dishes
Blackberries	Avocado, green	Brandy vinegar
Currants	Basil	Caviar
Dates, fresh	Chard	Chinese oyster sauce
Figs, fresh	Chives	Fish, meat, shrimp and shellfish*
Goji berries	Coriander	
Lemon zest	Green peppers	Kraft® Italian Dressing
Loganberry	Horseradish	
Papaya	Kelp	Kraft® Mayonnaise
Passion fruit	Oregano	Oils
Rhubarb	Parsnips	Kraft® Thousand Island Dressing®
	Peppermint, fresh	
	Rice	Pepper and salt
	Rosemary	Rice bread
	Rutabaga	Rice noodles
	Squash: Butternut, calabash, giant and spaghetti	Soy oil
	Thyme	Spelt flour
	Yam	Tabasco® sauce

*Non pureed and without breading and sauce.

Beverages	Other	
Black coffee	Baking powder	Pecan nuts
Brandy	Brazil nuts	Pine nuts
Gin	Brown sugar	Pistachios
Jasmine tea	Cashews	Pumpkin seeds
Maté tea	Coconut	Rice bread
Peppermint tea	Gelatin	Spelt
Rum	Ginkgo	Walnuts
Tequila	Licorice	White sugar
Tonic Water	Macadamia nuts	
Vodka	Maple syrup	
Water	Peanut butter	
Whiskey	Peanuts	

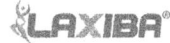

2.7 Recepies

2.7.1 Kiwi sauce (e.g. with ice)

What you need (one serving):

Three tsp. of maple syrup
Two ripe green kiwi fruits
Two tsp. of lime or lemon juice

Preparation:

Peel the kiwis, dice them and blend them afterwards together with the lime or lemon juice. If you love pure green, sieve out the remaining black seeds later on.

2.7.2 Lemon bar

What you need:
For the dough:

3/5 cup of butter
¾ cup of flour (celiac disease? Use gluten free flour)
One tbsp. milk
1/5 cup of g rice flour
4/5 cup of brown sugar

For the topping:

Three eggs
2 tbsp. of flour (celiac disease? Use gluten free flour)
Icing sugar
The zest of three lemons
4/5 cup of mL lemon juice
4/5 cup of sugar

Preparation:

Preheat the oven at 430 °f top and bottom heat or 390 °f air circulation. Cover a 9in baking tray with baking paper. Mix the butter, the flour, rice flour and sugar in a bowl, until only small lumps form. Then add the milk and spread the dough on the baking tray. Let it bake for 17 minutes until golden brown. Then remove the and reduce the oven temperature to 390 °f top and bottom heat or 360 °f air circulation. Whisk the lemon juice and the eggs, the sugar, the flour and the lemon zest in a bowl. Pour this concentrate over the dough and bake the lemon bars for another 15 minutes until the surface almost firm. Let it cool down on the tray. Finally, cut and powder - ready to enjoy.

2.7.3 Orange-peppermint-salad

What you need (for four servings)**:**

12 pitted dates, cut lengthwise
Four oranges
A small bunch of mint: some leaves finely cut and a few left a whole
One tbsp. of water

Preparation:

Peel the orange and place it together with the liberated juice in a bowl. Afterward, add the date pieces and the chopped peppermint leaves to the water and mix gently. Finally, top it with whole mint leaves.

2.7.4 Pancakes

What you need:

One egg
Half a cup of flour (celiac disease? Use gluten free flour)
1 and ¼ cup of rice milk
Sunflower oil

Preparation:

Put the flour into a bowl and make a hole in the middle, in which you put the egg together with the rice milk. Now whisk everything well with a mixer. Add a quarter of the rice milk and continue to add the rest once the batter is lump free. Now let the dough rest and after 20 minutes whisk it again. Preheat a small non-stick frying pan and pour the oil into it. Cover the whole bottom of the pan with a thin layer of dough. Fry the pancakes on each side, until golden brown. Place some baking paper between the pancakes when you pile them, so they remain crispy. Serve with any filling.

2.7.5 Pizza dough

What you need:

7g (one filled tsp) yeast (celiac disease? Use dry gluten-free yeast. First, let it rise with a tsp. of sugar in a cup that is half-full of water. After that, mix it with the rest of the water and flour. Often, it takes some time until the dough has risen.)
One and ½ cups of flour (celiac disease? Use gluten-free flour, here you may have to experiment a bit)
One 1/5 cups of water

Preparation:

Put the flour with a tsp. salt, yeast and 275 mL lukewarm water in a bowl and mix everything for about 5 minutes to form a dough. Now, take out the dough and let it rise it in a lightly oiled bowl until it rises about twice the size. Knead the dough afterwards for a bit, then cut it in half and roll out each of both parts on a thin layer of flour as thin as possible. Now garnish the pizza as desired and bake in the oven at 430 °f air circulation.

2.7.6 Rhubarb, roasted

What you need (five servings):
1 and 1/3 cup of Rhubarb
1/3 cup of brown sugar

Preparation:
Preheat the oven at 390 °f top and bottom heat or 360 °f air circulation. Wash the Rhubarb then shake off the water. Cut the end and the middle of the sticks into small finger-sized pieces. Cover a closed baking tray with a baking sheet and spread the Rhubarb on it. Sprinkle some sugar over it and cover the Rhubarb with it. Bake the Rhubarb for about 15 minutes with baking paper on top. Then remove the baking paper and shake the plate slightly. Then continue baking for about five minutes. When the Rhubarb is ready, it is soft, but not mushy.

2.7.7 Rhubarb cake

What you need:

One packet of baking powder (celiac disease? Use gluten-free baking powder)
Four large eggs
One cup of flour (celiac disease? Use gluten free flour)
Icing sugar
Pre-roasted Rhubarb, as described before.
One cup of sweet cream butter and even something for the baking tray
One tsp. vanilla extract
3/5 cup of custard
One cup of brown sugar

Preparation:

First, prepare the roasted Rhubarb and drain the juice. Preheat now the oven at 390 °f top and bottom heat or 180 degrees air circulation. Wipe a nine in cake springform pan with butter. Put 3 tbsp. of the vanilla pudding in a separate bowl. The rest you whisk up creamy with butter, the flour, baking powder, eggs and sugar in a bowl. Pour one-third of the mix in the cake form and place about half of the Rhubarb over it. Put one more third of dough over this layer and flatten it as smooth as possible. Cover the top with the rest of the Rhubarb and pour the remaining mixture over it, this time, the surface remains rough. Then use the remaining 3 tbsp. of the vanilla pudding to place on top. Bake the cake for 40 minutes, until it rises and becomes golden. Cover it with baking paper and leave it baking for another 15 minutes. The cake is ready when you stab it with a toothpick, and it comes out clean. Sprinkle some icing sugar over the cake after it cooled down.

2.7.8 Rucola salad

What you need (for 2-3 servings)**:**

Four tsp. vinegar from vinegar essence-water mixture
Two cups of grill cheese (e.g., halumi)
Three tbsp. of olive oil
Three medium, skinned oranges
One small bunch of chopped peppermint
3/5 cup of Rocket salad
1/5 cup (3 tbsp.) of roasted walnuts

Preparation:

Heat up a pan in which you fry the 1/3in sized grill cheese slices for about 1 to 2 minutes until they begin to melt. Mix the oranges with the juice from the peeling; the mint leaves and the vinegar gently in a bowl. Now add the walnuts and the rocket salad and mix well. Place the cheese slices on top. Finally, season the salad with black pepper - good appetite.

2.7.9 Spaghetti al salmone

What you need (for 2-3 portions)**:**

Two small finely ground chillies
Four tbsp. capers without the water from the glass
Two cloves of garlic
½ cup of mL extra virgin olive oil
4/5 cup of rocket salad
Two cups of spaghetti (celiac disease? Use gluten-free pasta)
200g salmon pieces
Two tbsp. of small cubes of white bread (celiac disease? Use gluten-free bread or go without croutons)
Lemon zest, meaning the yellow skin of a well-washed lemon

Preparation:

Heat up two tbsp. of olive oil in the pan and toast in the bread cubes over medium heat for three to four minutes, until golden brown. Place in a small bowl afterwards. Cook the spaghetti in salted water until al dente. Meanwhile, squeeze out the garlic cloves and heat the garlic with the chili powder and the remaining oil in the pan. Please make sure not to fry the garlic. Let the pasta drain and place them in a preheated bowl. Next, put the grated lemon zest and capers into the oil. Pour it over the pasta and spread it well. At last, you mix everything with the salmon and the rocket salad. Sprinkle the croutons over it before serving—et voila.

2.7.10 Sweet potato- or salami & pesto-pizza

What you need (for two servings):
3/5 cup of ciabatta bread-dough mixture
½ cup of mozzarella balls
Two tsp. Olive oil, one for pizza and one for the baking tray
Two tbsp. green pesto
A handful of rocket salad
4/9 cup of sweet potatoes (or salami)

Preparation:
Peel the potatoes, cut them into slices and boil them for 15 minutes in salted water. Then drain and let cool down briefly. Meanwhile, preheat the oven to 430 °f. Form the dough into a pizza shape and place it on a pre-oiled baking sheet. Now wait for 15 minutes. Spread the pesto on the pizza base. Sprinkle half of the mozzarella over it. The next layer is the potatoes (or salami) and on top of it is the rest of the mozzarella. Let the pizza bake for 15 to 18 minutes until the crust is golden brown and the cheese bubbles. Finally, put the rocket salad on the pizza and season with black pepper.

2.7.11 Thuna pizza

What you need (for eight servings):

A pack of cream cheese (225g)
2/3 cup of finely sliced mozzarella
Pepper
One and 2/3 cups (400g) pizza dough (celiac disease? Use gluten-free dough)
Small bunch chives
A can of tuna

Preparation:

Preheat the oven to 430 °f. Bake the dough briefly. Spread the cream cheese over it. Now cover the pizza base with tuna and mozzarella, season the pizza with pepper and finish baking. Meanwhile, wash the chives and cut it finely to spread it on the pizza, when it is ready.

2.7.12 Tropical fruit salad

What you need (six servings):

One and 2/3 cups of pieced cantaloupe
Two peeled kiwis
One and 2/3 cups of lychees
Three peeled oranges
Two stalks of lemongrass
1/3 cup of brown sugar

Preparation:

Cut the lemon grass into pieces and crush it with a rolling pin. Peel the lychees and remove the seeds, catch the juice. Mix the juice with the sugar and the lemongrass and heat it up for about a minute in a pan until the sugar has melted. Then let the broth cool down and sprinkle it over the fruits.

2.8 Stress management

Stress can affect your stomach and worsen sorbitol intolerance symptoms. Hence, it is important to reduce it. To find out its effect on you, fill out your symptom-test-sheet on a day when you have a lot of stress. Developing a solution-oriented way to manage your worries can help you do so. How does that help? The more you stress over something, the more brain areas that you need for a reasonable decision are being set off. The body does so, because, in a certain way, our bodies are prepared for an earlier historical era. Dangerous situations like an attack by a wolf pack left us with three options: fight, flight or playing dead. If we spent too much time thinking in such a situation, it was game over! Hence, we are poled to stop thinking as soon as we feel we are in danger—which is not always helpful in our modern time.

If nowadays your boss storms into your office with some tricky and pressing demands of a huge client, neither a spontaneous attack nor jumping out of the window or acting as dead will be recommendable. Seriously, nowadays usually much different factors trigger stress than it was a few thousand years ago. Aside from noise, extreme temperatures, and air pollution, it is especially the feeling of losing control in a situation, which feels threatening to us. Fear can grab you, when a project is particularly delicate and important, something fundamental has to change, and you are under time pressure.

At the advent of fear, the release of hormones supports fight and flight reactions that enable us to make quick, even if ill-conceived, decisions. Everything inside of you screams "Do something immidiately, no matter what!" Large parts of our brain are set aside for that purpose. You feel stress and tend to make impulsive rather than rational decisions. The hormones lead to a shut down of vast areas of your brain at that moment; you feel stress. The third option your mind conceives in a dangerous situation, playing dead, somewhat corresponds to the extreme modern-day phenomena that is widely known as burnout.

So you have the impulses of a Stone Age hunter but the tasks of a top manager: how can you make that fit together? The only option you have to resist your impulse is to take command of your body and mind. To react appropriately, you are required not to have your hormones to turn off your resources for rational decision-making.

Once your body feels in danger, it is a challenge to halt the rolling wheel of your body's emergency reactions abruptly. Hence, the best thing you can do is to prevent these stress reactions from evolving in the first place. Yoga and progressive muscle relaxation before work are useful stress preventers. Using such techniques before going to work is sensible, as it is seldom possible to take an hour off during the workday. Breaks and disruptions during your working hours are also **counterproductive** if you are dealing with complex tasks; they often lead to poor decisions, more stress, and a short temper. Thus, try to avoid disruption when dealing with sophisticated tasks. You will agree if you imagine working on a complex calculation while your phone is ringing and your colleague enters to chat with you and a technician wanting to maintain your printer is waiting in front of the door. Therefore, try to avoid distractions when you are dealing with challenging tasks.

However, interruptions of simple mental or physical labor lasting a few minutes, rather than seconds, result in slight positive effects. Taking breaks from hard physical labor, meanwhile, show even stronger benefits, lowering the risk of injuries and enhancing endurance. You do not want to be following a printer printing during your break. To make the best use of it, close your eyes and focus on your breathing. Whenever thoughts come up, focus your whole attention bad on your breath without evaluating the thoughts. What makes this better is counting the times that you breathe out and feeling your breath leave your mouth.

Still, relaxation alone might not be the solution. Often, you can identify general worries that effect your mood. So how do you deal with such concerns? Many try to evade them by trying to ignore them, distract themselves or even take alcohol or other supposed comforters. Instead of bringing you closer to your goal, such a reaction, makes matters worse in most cases. The only thing that will help you resolve your troublesome thoughts is actively dealing with them. Only if you can name them, you can find solutions. Also, consider this; ignorance may well be one of the leading causes of failure.

Of course, for most worries no one hands you the solution on a silver platter. You have to take action. An open examination of your concerns and the right strategy can lead you towards a feasible solution. There is an immediate positive effect of this, independent from what solution you find: you avoid panic actions that one tends to in charged situations. If you regularly call a spade a spade and rationally seek solutions to situations you worry about you reduce the number of poor decisions.

By doing so, you can even use your fears—through the process of conquering them—to help you become more successful in your everyday life. What I recommend you do is sit down at a quiet desk at the beginning or end of the day. Next, think about what you are worried about right now and which steps you need to take to prevent the feared outcomes.

It is helpful to create an Excel spreadsheet for doing so or to purchase the standardized and printer-optimized edition at *www.Laxiba.com*. If you want to create the table by yourself, call the first sheet "Worries" and the second one "Task List." Next, write down the following task headings in the first spreadsheet: "Current Worries," "Preventive Measure A," "Preventive Measure B" and "Preventive Measure C." Then enter the following column titles in the second spreadsheet: "Task," "Priority," "Deadline," "Who does it?" and "Done."

You should write down your concerns in the first column of the first sheet. Then, think about what you will need to do to prevent these worries from becoming a reality. Think of three alternatives for each outcome. Enter these into the "Preventive Measure A–C" fields next to each worry, A being the action you want to take first. Then, transfer "Preventive Measure A" to the "Task List" sheet. Next, prioritize the tasks by employing an adapted version of the "Eisenhower method," an organization technique that takes importance and urgency into account, from A to E:

Task is important	**A** *ction now*	**B** *etter do it soon*
Task is unimportant	**C** *hance to do the task if you completed all A and B duties.*	**D** *ull moment task*
E *fface, don't do task*	**Task is urgent**	**Postponable task**

In the order from A to D, you then execute your duties on a daily basis. The category E is for tasks that are ineffective and therefore, you leave it. Hence, you prevent worrying and free yourself from doubting whether you are currently doing the right thing. After assessing the tasks from A to D, you fill out the column "Deadline," into which you enter the date at which you want to accomplish the task. Furthermore, you either note "I" or the name of the person that you want to delegate the work to in the column "Who does it?" Finally, you tick off the cell in the column „Done", when you have finished the task.

Another important aspect is keeping your life balanced. A fulfilled family life and friendships also help to improve your stress resistance. To name an example: taking a healthy exercise is beneficial for all areas of your life. Brought to an extreme, though, let's say if you spend ten hours per day at a fitness center, this will take too much of your time away from your other areas—unless you are a personal trainer. The four quadrants of your life are like the four legs of a stool you sit on. Let us call it your life-stool. If each leg is just as long as the others and all are adequately thick, you will sit well and safe. In however you chop off some from one or more legs repeatedly and strengthen another leg, you will start to waggle—until at some point, there is a crack, and you land on your patoot. You have to avoid this "breakdown". Of course, I know that this is exactly the dilemma that burdens many people nowadays. You feel that you have to perform continuously in all areas. Fathers do not only have to work. They also have to spend time with their family. They ought to bring their children to the violin tuition. Then in the evening, they should foster their social contacts and engage in the summer festival of their city. Having a well-trained body is necessary for many. On top of that, you ideally are relaxed and well groomed. For woman and mothers, the expectations are just as high. They feel like they have to perform like men at work and still manage their family, organize the spare time and stay fit. Expectations appear to rise everywhere.

So do not get me wrong: keeping your life in a healthy balance means finding the **right** balance between those things that are important to you personally. It is not about which expectations others have concerning your life's quadrants! It is not about what the society expects from you. What is important is that you consider the key aspects of your individual life. In the table below these are work, relaxation, family and spare time. For you, the quadrants may be different. You set the priorities yourself. Free yourself as much as possible from the influence of the acknowledgment by others, follow the saying "great horses jump tight" and develop a healthy self-confidence and composure.

Instead of delivering an over-the-top performance in one area but lousy results in all others, you want to do at least a satisfying job in all sectors, to remain capable in the end. Which of the family, spare time, relaxation and work quadrants are important is up to you, along with the results you are aiming for with them, such as spending time with those closest to you, taking daily walks, pursuing your hobbies and getting your work done properly. Furthermore, it is important to resist basing your success on external measures. You should nourish a healthy self-confidence and serenity in yourself. Thus, you need to know when finished the task you are doing well enough. Some people get into time trouble because they over deliver on some tasks and then have little time left to take care of other important tasks, which then causes stress. Often it takes 80% of the time to improve on the last 20% of a job, so it pays off if you know if the last 20% are worth it.

Family: *Spend time with those closest to you*	**Relaxation:** *Go out for a walk on a daily basis*
Spare time: *Pursue your hobbies regularly*	**Work:** *Get your work done properly*

You can measure your progress about the four quadrants on a monthly basis on a scale of 1 (very good) to 7 (very poor). Always assign 7 points to the area that you are happiest with and other numbers to the remaining quadrants in relation to that one. Afterward, consider whether you want to make any changes to how you are approaching these areas of your life and how you can make those changes. You can also use the spreadsheet you created to manage your worries.

One final point on the topic of stress, even if it may seem trivial: be mindful of your mood, and try to stay upbeat! What you need to do that depends on you. Your mood only partially depends on circumstances. Sometimes simply deciding to be in a good mood can do more than most people realize. Everyone has a load of problems to carry, and it is easier to take it if you commit yourself to a positive outlook.

Do things that excite you as often as possible. Perform activities that contribute to what is most important to you. Is it your family? Then plan an excursion with your family! Is it a sport? Then ask someone to go jogging with you, for example. Consciously take the time to do those things that are close to your heart. Maybe you now object that you do not have time for that and that such self-serving activities would only lead to more stress. Try it out! I bet this qualitatively precious time will not incur losses but help you to mount every day with more tranquility. Plan your activities around what is most important to you in your life. What that means is obviously personal to you! It is your treasure, per se, so you have to dig it out yourself. *Abraham Lincoln* had this to say, to send you on your way: "That some achieve great success is proof to all that others can achieve it as well."

Summary

Stress can foster sorbitol intolerance symptoms. Increase your resistance to stress by training to use relaxation techniques, naming fears and worries, developing and noting down solution strategies and adding priorities to them. Make sure you keep your life in the right balance by trading-off between the areas that are important to you. Keep your eye on your goal.

2.9 General summary

1. What you are dealing with
If you have a sorbitol intolerance, sorbitol in food can irritate your gut. The symptoms occur because of your body's limited capacity to absorb sorbitol before it reaches the large intestine, where it causes the discomforts. A sorbitol intolerance is often a chronic but do not cause cancer. In most cases, following a fitting diet reduces the symptoms to an acceptable level.

2. Are you a unique case?
According to the *World Gastroenterology Organisation (WGO)*, up to one billion people have a dietary intolerance or IBS around the globe. In a way, you are lucky, as you can use this book to help you to reduce your symptoms.

3. Good reasons to follow this diet
An intolerance accompanies you for a long time, maybe for the rest of your life. If the diet works, it is far cheaper than medical treatment and sometimes even more efficient. Many medicines also have side effects. If the diet works for you, it will also lead to a general improvement in your wellbeing. You should find that you are ill less often, better able to concentrate, better at fulfilling social obligations, stronger at sports—your new diet can even enhance your love life!

4. Why you want to take the level test
Sensitivities differ in their severity. The fewer dietary restrictions you face, the more you save yourself the effort and can enjoy a more varied selection of food.

5. What you should pay attention to for the diet
Two things: First, adhere to your portion sizes, which you find in the tables in Chapter 3. Thus, only eat as much of sorbitol containing foods as your enzyme workers can handle. Second, eat in a balanced way see Chapter 2.1.4.

6. Dealing with setbacks

You have decided to change your diet and have made the first steps in that direction. Now, you have to stick to it. Moreover, that means to assess properly short-term setbacks. Rebounds are a part of any change process. What is important is that you get back up! The experience of meeting success after facing a blow will strengthen you immensely and ensure that you will be able to get back up even faster next time around. At some point, your experiences and successes will make it a habit for you to persevere and stick to your diet.

It may help you to set a time each Sunday to fill out the symptom test sheet—independent of the other tests. Doing this will remind you of your goal and let you break down the necessary steps toward it on a weekly basis. What is also important is that you become aware of the hurdles you will face. It will be hard to restrict yourself concerning the consumption of some foods that you have come to love. Particularly at the beginning, it will be unnerving to ask for dietary considerations as a dinner guest. Your nutrition plan will be new to others; you may feel criticized for your insistence on maintaining your new eating habits. Explain that you need to do it for the sake of your health. At the same time, express your appreciation for others' support. Moreover, try not giving dietary advice unless someone asks you for it — respecting the eating habits of others. They are more likely to accept yours in turn.

The adversary left for you to face is not standing next to you at the buffet and believes to know better what you can consume. The best captains are always standing ashore. The adversary is in your head and regularly cries "do it as you did it before. Before it was easier!" The influence of our old habits is often greater than we think. After a few days of tenacity, this caller has his big appearance. As soon, as our vigilance is lower he whispers in our ear "This is how you have always done it, and it has always been good, everything else is too exhaustive for you. Simply, show your adversary your weekly symptom test sheet--it works like garlic against vampires. It is the best mean to get rid of old habits, and form new ones! If you always readjust your heading—your diet to your goal, you will come close to it in the end. If you proceed like that, you have a good chance to win against the trigger and old habit imp.

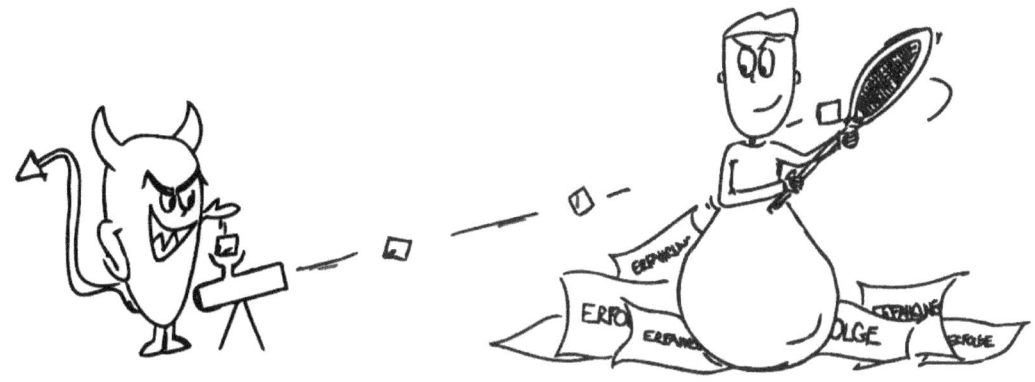

7. FAQs

What do you recommend concerning the diet? Drink at least 1.5 L of water every day. Eat a variety of foods. It is ok to eat foods that contain sorbitol, if your sensitivity level is low; you have to test that out for yourself, for example with the level test described in Chapter 4. To do even more for your health, work out regularly.

What can you do if a drink contains too much of sorbitol to drink a regular glass full? By diluting it with water, you can multiply your tolerable portion.

How can you save on cooking time? Cook larger portion sizes. Usually, it only takes a little longer than preparing small ones, and warming the food up is quick. You can keep rice and potatoes in the fridge for days, for instance. Purchase lockable glass containers to store your food keeping it fresh longer.

I have acute symptoms, what can I do? Take a walk and drink up to three liters of drinking water per day.

8. The LAXIBA® quickie

Be wary of diabetic, diet and light products, as well as dried fruit.

Do not start any diet without a proper diagnosis in advance. If you want to do something for your health, in general, stick to the advice see the Chapters starting on pages 35 and 67.

Feedback

Congratulations, you have mastered the background and strategy chapter. Around the globe, the brand *LAXIBA* represents an improved quality of life in connection with abdominal diseases and stress. Our goal is to offer you scientific solutions that you can implement swiftly to improve your life. To find out about our latest innovations, visit us at *https://laxiba.com* and register for our useletter.

Many improvements make this second edition the gold standard. Each contribution can help to make the book even better in the future. Thus, I am glad to learn about your experiences and your wishes! There are still grey areas, and regularly new foods enter the market that fit our tables well. To deal with the disease, it is important that you adapt your diet to the capacity of your enzyme workers. Therefore, we are interested in any food you are missing.

Would you like to take part in a coaching concerning the implementation of the diet or a workshop on stress management? We will have an offer that suits you. Visit us at *https://laxiba.com*. We look forward to getting to know you. Finally, I wish you prosperity, happiness and an improvement in your quality of life.

Your author,

J. N. Stratbucker – *John@Laxiba.com*

3

FOOD TABLES

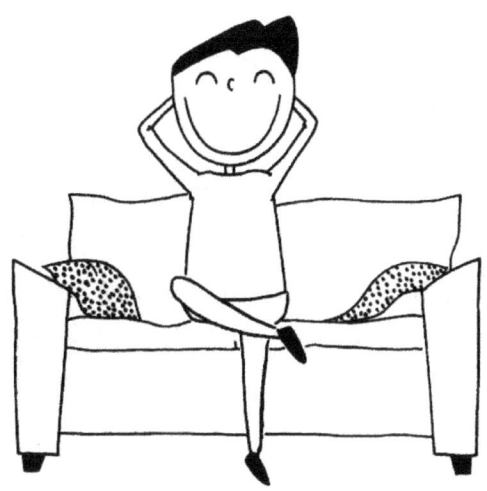

3.1 Introduction to the tables

In the following section, you will learn about the tolerable portion sizes for an intolerance towards sorbitol (the sum of nine sugar-alcohols). The statements all relate to **one meal**, assuming **three meals** per day and that only eat one food containing sorbitol. The stated amounts expect you to consume three meals per day, one at roughly 7 am, 1 pm and 7 pm, i.e., each with about **six hours** in between. However, the times are mainly just a reference point just make sure to keep the gaps! If you read the book carefully, you have also learned that eating in between the big meals can have a positive effect on your health. For each food, you can find out how much you can tolerate both in a suitable unit as well as in gram. These statements make cooking as well as eating out easy.

The lists are ordered by category. Apple juice is listed under beverages-juices, for example. The idea behind this is that you can easily find alternatives should your tolerated amount be small. At the end of the tables, you also find a food index, though, see page 207, which you can use if you are solely interested in finding out how much watermelon you can stomach.

The tables are set up in a manner that is easy to understand. Each page contains about 14 foods. In the tables, you find the category title in the first cell of each table. Below it, you can see the food names and next to them the tolerated amount explained by a proper unit or a smiley. Afterward, you find an explanation as well as the amount in gram.

It is important to us that the data quality is excellent. All figures originate from an analysis conducted by the *University of Minnesota*. For the first time, all nine sugar-alcohols to determine the sorbitol portion sizes to allow for a more reliable diet. In the following the symbols and units will be explained further.

Note: **Even if you stick to the standard portion sizes in the following tables, look at the low sensitivity amount as well. If the amount there is high, you can probably tolerate the food, because the standard portion sizes mean that you completely avoid sorbitol.**

3.1.1 Your personal sensitivity levels

Level 1 multiplier and sorbitol amount per meal by level

	Level	g	Table amount multiplier	Your level
Sorbitol and other sugar alcohols g/meal	Standard	0	×0	
	1	0.1	base	
	2	0.4	×4	
	3	0.7	×7	

The low sensitivity amount column in the tables refers to tolerance level 1 and the standard amount to level 0.

3.1.2 Explanation of the symbols

Here you will find an explanation of the symbols. The symbols show you at a glance how many units you can tolerate of the respective food. If you can see a smiley in the list, you will not find an amount. If the smiley looks sad, you should avoid the product if you have a sorbitol intolerance. If it smiles, you can enjoy it to your heart's content—if there is a big smile, it is completely free of sugar-alcohols.

Symbol	Meaning
	An average sized potion
	Slice(s)
	Piece(s)
	Hand(s) full
	Tablespoon(s)
	Bar
	Pinch
	Cup, 150 mL
	Glass, 200 mL
	Avoid the consumption. You can tolerate less than ¼ of the lowest amount due to the high sorbitol load of the food.
	Nearly free of sorbitol. You are likely to tolerate the food well.
	Free consumption as the food is free of sorbitol.

3.1.3 Explanation of the statements

Label	Meaning
Standard amount	In this column, you find the name of the unit or the meaning of the smiley. Behind it, in brackets, is stated how much gram one unit has followed by the tolerated amount per meal in total.
¼, ½, ¾, 1, 1¼, 1½, 1¾, 2, etc.	The tolerated amount of the respective unit, e.g., "cookie ½ piece" means you tolerate half a cookie of the type per meal, and "soup 1¾ portion" means one and three-fourths of a portion of the soup.
Avoid consumption.	Avoid the consumption of the food; it contains much of sorbitol.
Avoid consumption!	Avoid the consumption of the food; it contains very much of sorbitol.
Avoid consumption!!	Avoid the consumption of the food; it contains an extreme load of sorbitol.

Note: Please always look at the ingredients as stated on the food packages as well. Especially, if the list does not mention a producer, the composition may vary. In addition, you should consider the weight of one unit in gram. The average portion sizes underlying the statements may be larger or smaller than you expect. For example, 30g of some cereals can fill an entire bowl while you can eat 30g of a brownie in three bites. If you suffer from a fructose intolerance only, it is sufficient to base your consumption decisions on the fructose portions only, as the sorbitol has been accounted for here already.

CATEGORY LIST-INDEX

3.2	**Athletes**	**83**
3.3	**Beverages**	**85**
3.3.1	Alcoholic	85
3.3.2	Hot beverages	91
3.3.3	Juices	95
3.3.4	Other beverages	98
3.4	**Cold dishes**	**101**
3.4.1	Bread	101
3.4.2	Cereals	103
3.4.3	Cold cut	106
3.4.4	Dairy products	110
3.4.5	Nuts and snacks	115
3.4.6	Sweet pastries	118
3.4.7	Sweets	123
3.5	**Warm dishes**	**128**
3.5.1	Meals	128
3.5.2	Meat and fish	133
3.5.3	Side dishes	136
3.6	**Fast food chains**	**138**
3.6.1	Burger King®	138
3.6.2	KFC®	140
3.6.3	McDonald's®	141
3.6.4	Subway®	143
3.6.5	Taco Bell®	145
3.6.6	Wendy's®	146
3.7	**Fruits and vegetables**	**147**
3.7.1	Fruit	147
3.7.2	Vegetables	152
3.8	**Ice cream**	**159**
3.9	**Ingredients**	**162**

3.2 Athletes

Athletes	Sorbitol standard		SORBITOL Low sensitivity amount	
Clif Bar®, Chocolate Chip	☹	Avoid	2¼	Piece (68g); 153g in total.
Clif Bar®, Crunchy Peanut Butter	☹	Avoid	2½	Piece (68g); 170g in total.
Clif Bar®, Oatmeal Raisin Walnut	☹	Avoid	1¾	Piece (68g); 119g in total.
Electrolyte replacement drink	☺	Free	☺	Free of sorbitol.
Gatorade®, all flavors	☺	Free	☺	Free of sorbitol.
Gatorade®, from dry mix, all flavors	☺	Free	☺	Free of sorbitol.
Glaceau® Vitaminwater 10	☹	Avoid	☹	Avoid consumption!!
Glaceau® Vitaminwater Energy	☺	Free	☺	Free of sorbitol.
Glaceau® Vitaminwater Essential	☺	Free	☺	Free of sorbitol.
Glaceau® Vitaminwater Focus	☺	Free	☺	Free of sorbitol.
Glaceau® Vitaminwater Power-C	☺	Free	☺	Free of sorbitol.
Glaceau® Vitaminwater Revive	☺	Free	☺	Free of sorbitol.
High-protein Bar, generic	☹	Avoid	76¾	Piece (65g); 4989g in total.
Power Bar® 20g Protein Plus, Chocolate Crisp	☹	Avoid	☹	Avoid consumption!!
Power Bar® 20g Protein Plus, Chocolate Peanut Butter	☹	Avoid	☹	Avoid consumption!!

Athletes	SORBITOL Stand.		SORBITOL Low sensitivity amount	
Power Bar® 30g Protein Plus, Chocolate Brownie	☺	Nearly free	☺	Nearly free of sorbitol
Power Bar® Harvest Energy®, Double Chocolate Crisp	☹	Avoid 10¾	🍰	Piece (65g); 699g in total.
Power Bar® Performance Energy®, Banana	☺	Nearly free	☺	Nearly free of sorbitol
Power Bar® Performance Energy®, Chocolate	☹	Avoid 76¾	🍰	Piece (65g); 4989g in total.
Power Bar® Performance Energy®, Cookie Dough	☺	Nearly free	☺	Nearly free of sorbitol
Power Bar® Performance Energy®, Mixed Berry Blast	☹	Avoid 19	🍰	Piece (65g); 1235g in total.
Power Bar® Performance Energy®, Vanilla Crisp	☺	Nearly free	☺	Nearly free of sorbitol
Powerade®, all flavors	☺	Free	☺	Free of sorbitol.

3.3 Beverages

3.3.1 Alcoholic

Alcoholic	SORBITOL Stand.		SORBITOL Low sensitivity amount	
Ale	☹ Avoid	10	Glass (200g); 2000 mL in total.
Amaretto	☹ Avoid	¼	Glass (200g); 50 mL in total.
Apple juice or cider, made from frozen	☹ Avoid	☹	Avoid consumption!
Applejack liquor	☺ Free	☺	Free of sorbitol.
Aquavit	☺ Free	☺	Free of sorbitol.
Beer	☹ Avoid	10	Glass (200g); 2000 mL in total.
Beer, low alcohol	☺ Free	☺	Free of sorbitol.
Beer, low carb	☹ Avoid	10	Glass (200g); 2000 mL in total.
Beer, non alcoholic	☺ Free	☺	Free of sorbitol.
Black Russian	☹ Avoid	8¼	Glass (200g); 1650 mL in total.
Bloody Mary	☹ Avoid	½	Glass (200g); 100 mL in total.
Bourbon	☺ Free	☺	Free of sorbitol.
Brandy	☺ Free	☺	Free of sorbitol.
Brandy, flavored	☹ Avoid	¼	Glass (200g); 50 mL in total.

Alcoholic	SORBITOL Stand.		SORBITOL Low sensitivity amount	
Burgundy wine, red	☹	Avoid	½	Glass (200g); 100 mL in total.
Burgundy wine, white	☹	Avoid	¾	Glass (200g); 150 mL in total.
Campari®	☹	Avoid	¼	Glass (200g); 50 mL in total.
Cape Cod	☹	Avoid	25	Glass (200g); 5000 mL in total.
Champagne punch	☹	Avoid	1	Glass (200g); 200 mL in total.
Champagne, white	☹	Avoid	¾	Glass (200g); 150 mL in total.
Chardonnay	☹	Avoid	¾	Glass (200g); 150 mL in total.
Club soda	☺	Free	☺	Free of sorbitol.
Cognac	☺	Free	☺	Free of sorbitol.
Cointreau®	☹	Avoid	¼	Glass (200g); 50 mL in total.
Creme de Cocoa	☹	Avoid	2½	Glass (200g); 500 mL in total.
Creme de menthe	☹	Avoid	¼	Glass (200g); 50 mL in total.
Curacao	☹	Avoid	¼	Glass (200g); 50 mL in total.
Daiquiri	☺	Free	☺	Free of sorbitol.
Eggnog, regular	☺	Free	☺	Free of sorbitol.
Fruit punch, alcoholic	☹	Avoid	1	Glass (200g); 200 mL in total.

Alcoholic	SORBITOL Stand.		SORBITOL Low sensitivity amount	
Gibson	Avoid	3¼	Glass (200g); 650 mL in total.
Gin	Free		Free of sorbitol.
Grand Marnier®	Avoid	¼	Glass (200g); 50 mL in total.
Grasshopper	Avoid	¾	Glass (200g); 150 mL in total.
Harvey Wallbanger	Avoid	¼	Glass (200g); 50 mL in total.
Kamikaze	Avoid	1	Glass (200g); 200 mL in total.
Kirsch	Avoid	¼	Glass (200g); 50 mL in total.
Light beer	Avoid	12½	Glass (200g); 2500 mL in total.
Liqueur, coffee flavored	Avoid	2½	Glass (200g); 500 mL in total.
Long Island iced tea	Avoid	16½	Glass (200g); 3300 mL in total.
Mai Tai	Avoid	1¾	Glass (200g); 350 mL in total.
Malt liquor	Avoid	10	Glass (200g); 2000 mL in total.
Manhattan	Avoid	2	Glass (200g); 400 mL in total.
Margarita, frozen	Avoid	7	Glass (200g); 1400 mL in total.
Martini®	Avoid	3¼	Glass (200g); 650 mL in total.
Merlot, red	Avoid	½	Glass (200g); 100 mL in total.

Alcoholic	SORBITOL Stand.		SORBITOL Low sensitivity amount	
Merlot, white	☺	Free	☺	Free of sorbitol.
Mint Julep	☺	Free	☺	Free of sorbitol.
Mojito	☺	Free	☺	Free of sorbitol.
Muscatel	☹	Avoid	½	Glass (200g); 100 mL in total.
Non-alcoholic wine	☹	Avoid	50	Glass (200g); 10000 mL in total.
Ouzo	☹	Avoid	¼	Glass (200g); 50 mL in total.
Pina colada	☹	Avoid	4	Glass (200g); 800 mL in total.
Port wine	☹	Avoid	½	Glass (200g); 100 mL in total.
Riesling	☹	Avoid	¾	Glass (200g); 150 mL in total.
Rob Roy	☹	Avoid	2½	Glass (200g); 500 mL in total.
Rompope (eggnog with alcohol)	☺	Free	☺	Free of sorbitol.
Root beer	☺	Free	☺	Free of sorbitol.
Rose wine, other types	☺	Free	☺	Free of sorbitol.
Rum	☺	Free	☺	Free of sorbitol.
Rum and cola	☺	Free	☺	Free of sorbitol.
Rusty nail	☹	Avoid	¾	Glass (200g); 150 mL in total.

Alcoholic	SORBITOL Stand.	SORBITOL Low sensitivity amount	
Sake	Avoid	½	Glass (200g); 100 mL in total.
Sambuca	Avoid	¼	Glass (200g); 50 mL in total.
Sangria	Avoid	¾	Glass (200g); 150 mL in total.
Schnapps, all flavors	Avoid	½	Glass (200g); 100 mL in total.
Scotch and soda	Free		Free of sorbitol.
Screwdriver	Avoid	¼	Glass (200g); 50 mL in total.
Seabreeze	Avoid	2½	Glass (200g); 500 mL in total.
Singapore sling	Avoid	4½	Glass (200g); 900 mL in total.
Sloe gin	Avoid	¼	Glass (200g); 50 mL in total.
Sloe gin fizz	Avoid	1½	Glass (200g); 300 mL in total.
Southern Comfort®	Free		Free of sorbitol.
Sylvaner	Avoid	¾	Glass (200g); 150 mL in total.
Tequila	Free		Free of sorbitol.
Tequila sunrise	Avoid	3¼	Glass (200g); 650 mL in total.
Tokaji Wine	Avoid	½	Glass (200g); 100 mL in total.
Tom Collins	Avoid	16½	Glass (200g); 3300 mL in total.

Alcoholic	SORBITOL Stand.		SORBITOL Low sensitivity amount	
Triple Sec	☹	Avoid	¼	Glass (200g); 50 mL in total.
Vodka	☺	Free	☺	Free of sorbitol.
Whiskey	☺	Free	☺	Free of sorbitol.
Whiskey sour	☹	Avoid	6¼	Glass (200g); 1250 mL in total.
White Russian	☹	Avoid	8¼	Glass (200g); 1650 mL in total.
Wine spritzer	☹	Avoid	1	Glass (200g); 200 mL in total.

3.3.2 Hot beverages

Hot beverages	SORBITOL Stand.		SORBITOL Low sensitivity amount	
Americano, decaf, without flavored syrup	😊 Free		😊 Free of sorbitol.	
Americano, with flavored syrup	😊 Free		😊 Free of sorbitol.	
Americano, without flavored syrup	😊 Free		😊 Free of sorbitol.	
Brown sugar	😊 Free		😊 Free of sorbitol.	
Cafe au lait, without flavored syrup	😊 Free		😊 Free of sorbitol.	
Cafe latte, with flavored syrup	😊 Free		😊 Free of sorbitol.	
Cafe latte, without flavored syrup	😊 Free		😊 Free of sorbitol.	
Camomile tea	😊 Free		😊 Free of sorbitol.	
Cappuccino, bottled or canned	😊 Free		😊 Free of sorbitol.	
Cappuccino, decaf, with flavored syrup	😊 Free		😊 Free of sorbitol.	
Cappuccino, decaf, without flavored syrup	😊 Free		😊 Free of sorbitol.	
Chai tea	😊 Free		😊 Free of sorbitol.	
Chicory coffee	☹ Avoid		11 ☕ Cup (150g); 1650 mL in total.	
Coffee substitute, prepared	😊 Free		😊 Free of sorbitol.	
Coffee, prepared from flavored mix, sugar free	☹ Avoid		66½ ☕ Cup (150g); 9975 mL in total.	

Hot beverages	SORBITOL Stand.		SORBITOL Low sensitivity amount	
Dandelion tea	☺	Free	☺	Free of sorbitol.
Demitasse	☺	Free	☺	Free of sorbitol.
Dove® Promises, Milk Chocolate	☺	Free	☺	Free of sorbitol.
Earl Grey, strong	☺	Free	☺	Free of sorbitol.
Espresso, without flavored syrup	☺	Free	☺	Free of sorbitol.
Evaporated milk, diluted, skim (fat free)	☺	Free	☺	Free of sorbitol.
Fennel tea	☺	Free	☺	Free of sorbitol.
Frappuccino®	☺	Free	☺	Free of sorbitol.
Frappuccino®, bottled or canned	☺	Free	☺	Free of sorbitol.
Frappuccino®, bottled or canned, light	☺	Free	☺	Free of sorbitol.
Green tea, strong	☺	Free	☺	Free of sorbitol.
Herbal tea	☺	Free	☺	Free of sorbitol.
Hershey's® Bliss Hot Drink White Chocolate, prepared	☺	Free	☺	Free of sorbitol.
Hot chocolate, homemade	☹	Avoid	66½ ☕	Cup (150g); 9975 mL in total.
Instant coffee mix, unprepared	☹	Avoid	☹	Avoid consumption!
Irish coffee with alcohol and whipped cream	☺	Free	☺	Free of sorbitol.

Hot beverages	SORBITOL Stand.		SORBITOL Low sensitivity amount	
Jasmine tea	☺	Free	Free of sorbitol.	
Light cream	☺	Free	Free of sorbitol.	
Milk, lactose reduced Lactaid®, skim (fat free)	☺	Free	Free of sorbitol.	
Milk, lactose reduced Lactaid®, whole	☺	Free	Free of sorbitol.	
Milk, unprepared dry powder, nonfat, instant	☺	Free	Free of sorbitol.	
Mocha, without flavored syrup	☺	Free	Free of sorbitol.	
Nestle® Hot Cocoa Dark Chocolate, prepared	☺	Nearly free	Nearly free of sorbitol	
Nestle® Hot Cocoa Rich Milk Chocolate, prepared	☺	Free	Free of sorbitol.	
Oolong tea	☺	Free	Free of sorbitol.	
Soy milk, chocolate, sugar, not fortified, ready-to-drink	☹	Avoid	4¼	Cup (150g); 638 mL in total.
Splenda®	☺	Free	Free of sorbitol.	
Starbucks® Hot Cocoa Double Chocolate, prepared	☹	Avoid	66½	Cup (150g); 9975 mL in total.
Starbucks® Hot Cocoa Salted Caramel, prepared	☹	Avoid	66½	Cup (150g); 9975 mL in total.
Sugar, white granulated	☺	Free	Free of sorbitol.	
Sweetened condensed milk	☺	Free	Free of sorbitol.	
Sweetened condensed milk, reduced fat	☺	Free	Free of sorbitol.	

Hot beverages	SORBITOL Stand.		SORBITOL Low sensitivity amount	
Swiss Miss® Hot Cocoa Sensible Sweets Diet, sugar free, prepared	☺	Free	☺	Free of sorbitol.
Whipped cream, aerosol	☺	Free	☺	Free of sorbitol.
Whipped cream, aerosol, fat free	☺	Free	☺	Free of sorbitol.
White tea	☺	Free	☺	Free of sorbitol.
Zsweet®	☹	Avoid	☹	Avoid consumption!!

3.3.3 Juices

Juices	SORBITOL Stand.		SORBITOL Low sensitivity amount
Apple banana strawberry juice	Avoid		Avoid consumption!
Apple grape juice	Avoid		Avoid consumption!
Apricot nectar	Avoid	¼	Glass (200g); 50 mL in total.
Arby's® orange juice	Avoid	¼	Glass (200g); 50 mL in total.
Black cherry juice	Avoid	2½	Glass (200g); 500 mL in total.
Black currant juice	Avoid	1½	Glass (200g); 300 mL in total.
Blackberry juice	Free		Free of sorbitol.
Capri Sun®, all flavors	Avoid	2	Glass (200g); 400 mL in total.
Carrot juice	Avoid	4	Glass (200g); 800 mL in total.
Cranberry juice cocktail, with apple juice	Avoid		Avoid consumption!
Cranberry juice cocktail, with blueberry juice	Avoid		Avoid consumption!
Fruit drink or punch, ready to drink	Avoid	2	Glass (200g); 400 mL in total.
Grapefruit juice, unsweetened, white	Avoid	¼	Glass (200g); 50 mL in total.
Kern's® Mango-Orange Nectar	Avoid	2	Glass (200g); 400 mL in total.
Kern's® Strawberry Nectar	Avoid	¾	Glass (200g); 150 mL in total.

Juices	SORBITOL Stand.		SORBITOL Low sensitivity amount	
Lemon juice, fresh	☹	Avoid	1½	Glass (200g); 300 mL in total.
Libby's® Apricot Nectar	☹	Avoid	¼	Glass (200g); 50 mL in total.
Libby's® Banana Nectar	☹	Avoid	25	Glass (200g); 5000 mL in total.
Libby's® Juicy Juice®, Apple Grape	☹	Avoid	¼	Glass (200g); 50 mL in total.
Libby's® Juicy Juice®, Grape	☹	Avoid	¼	Glass (200g); 50 mL in total.
Libby's® Pear Nectar	☹	Avoid	☹	Avoid consumption!
Lime juice, fresh	☺	Free	☺	Free of sorbitol.
Mango nectar	☹	Avoid	1¼	Glass (200g); 250 mL in total.
Northland® Cranberry Juice, all flavors	☹	Avoid	25	Glass (200g); 5000 mL in total.
Orange kiwi passion juice	☹	Avoid	¾	Glass (200g); 150 mL in total.
Passion fruit juice	☺	Free	☺	Free of sorbitol.
Peach juice	☹	Avoid	¾	Glass (200g); 150 mL in total.
Pear juice	☹	Avoid	☹	Avoid consumption!!
Pineapple juice	☹	Avoid	1¾	Glass (200g); 350 mL in total.
Pineapple orange drink	☺	Free	☺	Free of sorbitol.
Pomegranate juice	☹	Avoid	☹	Avoid consumption!

Juices	SORBITOL Stand.		SORBITOL Low sensitivity amount	
Raspberry juice	☹ Avoid		☹	Avoid consumption!
Tomato juice	☹ Avoid	¼		Glass (200g); 50 mL in total.
V-8® 100% A-C-E Vitamin Rich Vegetable Juice	☹ Avoid	3		Glass (200g); 600 mL in total.
Veryfine Cranberry Raspberry	☹ Avoid		☹	Avoid consumption!

3.3.4 Other beverages

Other beverages	SORBITOL Stand.	SORBITOL Low sensitivity amount
7 UP®	😊 Free	😊 Free of sorbitol.
Canfield's® Root Beer	😊 Free	😊 Free of sorbitol.
Canfield's® Root Beer, diet	😊 Free	😊 Free of sorbitol.
Cherry Coke®	😊 Free	😊 Free of sorbitol.
Coke Zero®	😊 Free	😊 Free of sorbitol.
Coke®	😊 Free	😊 Free of sorbitol.
Coke® with Lime	😊 Free	😊 Free of sorbitol.
Diet 7 UP®	😊 Free	😊 Free of sorbitol.
Diet Coke®	😊 Free	😊 Free of sorbitol.
Diet Dr. Pepper®	😊 Free	😊 Free of sorbitol.
Diet Pepsi®, fountain	😊 Free	😊 Free of sorbitol.
Fanta Zero®, fruit flavors	😊 Free	😊 Free of sorbitol.
Fanta® Red	😊 Free	😊 Free of sorbitol.
Fanta®, fruit flavors	😊 Free	😊 Free of sorbitol.
Ginger ale	😊 Free	😊 Free of sorbitol.

Other beverages	SORBITOL Stand.		SORBITOL Low sensitivity amount	
Lipton® Iced Tea Mix, with sugar, prepared	☺	Free	☺	Free of sorbitol.
Lipton® Instant 100% Tea, unsweetened, prepared	☺	Free	☺	Free of sorbitol.
Mineral Water	☺	Free	☺	Free of sorbitol.
Monster® Energy®	☺	Free	☺	Free of sorbitol.
Monster® Khaos	☹	Avoid	¼	Portion (240g); 60g in total.
Mountain Dew®	☺	Free	☺	Free of sorbitol.
Mountain Dew® Code Red	☺	Free	☺	Free of sorbitol.
Nestea® 100% Tea, unsweetened, dry	☺	Free	☺	Free of sorbitol.
Nestea® Iced Tea, Sugar Free, dry	☺	Free	☺	Free of sorbitol.
Nestea® Iced Tea, Sugar Free, prepared	☺	Free	☺	Free of sorbitol.
Nestea® Iced Tea, sweetened with sugar, dry	☺	Free	☺	Free of sorbitol.
No Fear®	☹	Avoid	50	Glass (200g); 10000 mL in total.
No Fear® Sugar Free	☺	Free	☺	Free of sorbitol.
Pepsi®	☺	Free	☺	Free of sorbitol.
Pepsi® Max	☺	Free	☺	Free of sorbitol.
Pepsi® Twist	☺	Free	☺	Free of sorbitol.

Other beverages	SORBITOL Stand.		SORBITOL Low sensitivity amount
Red Bull® Energy Drink	☺ Free		☺ Free of sorbitol.
Red Bull® Energy Drink Sugar Free	☺ Free		☺ Free of sorbitol.
Rockstar Original®	☹ Avoid	5	Glass (200g); 1000 mL in total.
Rockstar Original® Sugar Free	☹ Avoid	5	Glass (200g); 1000 mL in total.
Schweppes® Bitter Lemon	☺ Free		☺ Free of sorbitol.
Spearmint tea	☺ Free		☺ Free of sorbitol.
Sprite®	☺ Free		☺ Free of sorbitol.
Sprite® Zero	☺ Free		☺ Free of sorbitol.
Tap water	☺ Free		☺ Free of sorbitol.
Tonic water	☺ Free		☺ Free of sorbitol.
Tonic water, diet	☺ Free		☺ Free of sorbitol.
Vanilla Coke®	☺ Free		☺ Free of sorbitol.
Yerba® Mate tea	☺ Free		☺ Free of sorbitol.

3.4 Cold dishes

3.4.1 Bread

Bread	SORBITOL Stand.		SORBITOL Low sensitivity amount	
Baguette	☺	Free	☺	Free of sorbitol.
Cracked wheat bread, with raisins	☹	Avoid 4¼	☺	Slice (42g); 179g in total.
English muffin bread	☺	Free	☺	Free of sorbitol.
Focaccia bread	☺	Free	☺	Free of sorbitol.
French or Vienna roll	☺	Free	☺	Free of sorbitol.
GG® Scandinavian Bran Crispbread (Health Valley®)	☺	Free	☺	Free of sorbitol.
Gluten free bread	☺	Free	☺	Free of sorbitol.
Newman's Own® Organic Pretzels, Spelt	☺	Free	☺	Free of sorbitol.
Potato bread	☺	Nearly free	☺	Nearly free of sorbitol
Pumpernickel roll	☺	Free	☺	Free of sorbitol.
Rice bread	☺	Free	☺	Free of sorbitol.
Rye bread	☺	Free	☺	Free of sorbitol.
Rye roll	☺	Free	☺	Free of sorbitol.
Sourdough bread	☺	Free	☺	Free of sorbitol.

Bread	SORBITOL Stand.		SORBITOL Low sensitivity amount	
Soy bread	☹	Avoid	2	Slice (42g); 84g in total.
Toast, cinnamon and sugar, whole wheat bread	☺	Free	☺	Free of sorbitol.
Toast, wheat bread, with butter	☺	Free	☺	Free of sorbitol.
Triticale bread	☺	Free	☺	Free of sorbitol.
White bread, store bought	☺	Free	☺	Free of sorbitol.
White whole grain wheat bread	☹	Avoid	26¼	Slice (42g); 1103g in total.
Whole wheat bread, store bought	☺	Free	☺	Free of sorbitol.

3.4.2 Cereals

Cereals	SORBITOL Stand.		SORBITOL Low sensitivity amount	
All-Bran® Original (Kellogg's®)	Free			Free of sorbitol.
Amaranth Flakes (Arrowhead Mills)	Avoid	2½		Portion (30g); 75g in total.
Cascadian Farm® Organic Granola Bar, Trail Mix Dark Chocolate Cranberry	Avoid	71¼		Piece (35g); 2494g in total.
Cheerios® Snack Mix, all flavors	Nearly free			Nearly free of sorbitol
Chocolate Chex® (General Mills®)	Nearly free			Nearly free of sorbitol
Cinnamon toast crunch® (General Mills®)	Free			Free of sorbitol.
Cinnamon Toasters® (Malt-O-Meal®)	Free			Free of sorbitol.
Cocoa Krispies® (Kellogg's®)	Nearly free			Nearly free of sorbitol
Cocoa Puffs® (General Mills®)	Nearly free			Nearly free of sorbitol
Corn Chex® (General Mills®)	Nearly free			Nearly free of sorbitol
Corn Flakes (Kellogg's®)	Nearly free			Nearly free of sorbitol
Crunchy Nut Roasted Nut & Honey (Kellogg's®)	Avoid	15		Portion (30g); 450g in total.
Essentials Oat Bran cereal (Quaker®)	Free			Free of sorbitol.
Evaporated milk, diluted, skim (fat free)	Free			Free of sorbitol.
Familia Swiss Muesli®, Original Recipe	Avoid	1		Portion (55g); 55g in total.

Cereals	SORBITOL Stand.		SORBITOL Low sensitivity amount	
Fiber One Original® (General Mills®)	☺	Free	☺	Free of sorbitol.
Fiber One® Nutty Clusters & Almonds (General Mills®)	☺	Free	☺	Free of sorbitol.
Froot Loops® (Kellogg's®)	☺	Free	☺	Free of sorbitol.
Frosted Flakes® (Kellogg's®)	☺	Nearly free	☺	Nearly free of sorbitol
Frosted Flakes® Reduced Sugar (Kellogg's®)	☺	Nearly free	☺	Nearly free of sorbitol
Frosted Mini-Wheats Big Bite® (Kellogg's®)	☺	Free	☺	Free of sorbitol.
GoLEAN® Crisp! Cereal, Cinnamon Crumble (Kashi®)	☹	Avoid	25¾	Portion (55g); 1416g in total.
GoLEAN® Crunch! Cereal, Honey Almond Flax (Kashi®)	☹	Avoid	18	Portion (55g); 990g in total.
Health Valley® Multigrain Granola Bar, Chocolate Chip	☺	Nearly free	☺	Nearly free of sorbitol
Honey	☹	Avoid	1¾	Tbsp. (15g); 26g in total.
Honey Nut Chex® (General Mills®)	☹	Avoid	37	Portion (30g); 1110g in total.
Honey Smacks® (Kellogg's®)	☹	Avoid	83¼	Portion (30g); 2498g in total.
Kashi® Chewy Granola Bar, Cherry Dark Chocolate	☹	Avoid	1	Piece (35g); 35g in total.
Maple syrup, pure	☺	Free	☺	Free of sorbitol.
Milk, lactose reduced Lactaid®, skim (fat free) fortified with calcium or not	☺	Free	☺	Free of sorbitol.

Cereals	SORBITOL Stand.		SORBITOL Low sensitivity amount		
Mueslix® (Kellogg's®)		Avoid	2¾		Portion (55g); 151g in total.
Rice Krispies® (Kellogg's®)		Free			Free of sorbitol.
Sorghum		Free			Free of sorbitol.
Special K® Blueberry cereal (Kellogg's®)		Avoid	15		Portion (30g); 450g in total.
Special K® Cinnamon Pecan cereal (Kellogg's®)		Free			Free of sorbitol.
Special K® Original cereal (Kellogg's®)		Free			Free of sorbitol.
Special K® Red Berries cereal (Kellogg's®)		Avoid	41½		Portion (30g); 1245g in total.
Sprinkles Cookie Crisp® (General Mills®)		Nearly free			Nearly free of sorbitol.
Sunbelt Bakery® Chewy Granola Bar, Banana Harvest		Avoid	¾		Piece (25g); 19g in total.
Sunbelt Bakery® Granola Bar, Blueberry Harvest		Avoid	¾		Piece (25g); 19g in total.
Sunbelt Bakery® Chewy Granola Bar, Golden Almond		Avoid			Avoid consumption!
Sunbelt Bakery® Granola Bar, Low Fat Oatmeal Raisin		Avoid			Avoid consumption!
Sunbelt Bakery® Chewy Granola Bar, Oats & Honey		Avoid			Avoid consumption!
Sunbelt Bakery® Fudge Dipped Granola Bar, Coconut		Avoid			Avoid consumption!
Weetabix® Organic Crispy Flakes & Fiber		Free			Free of sorbitol.
Wheaties® (General Mills®)		Free			Free of sorbitol.

3.4.3 Cold cut

Cold cut	SORBITOL Stand.		SORBITOL Low sensitivity amount	
Almond butter, salted	☺	Free	☺	Free of sorbitol.
Almond butter, unsalted	☺	Free	☺	Free of sorbitol.
Alpine Lace 25% Reduced Fat, Mozzarella	☺	Free	☺	Free of sorbitol.
American cheese, processed	☺	Free	☺	Free of sorbitol.
Blue cheese	☺	Free	☺	Free of sorbitol.
Bologna, beef ring	☺	Free	☺	Free of sorbitol.
Bologna, combination of meats, light (reduced fat)	☺	Free	☺	Free of sorbitol.
Brie cheese	☺	Free	☺	Free of sorbitol.
Butter, light, salted	☺	Free	☺	Free of sorbitol.
Butter, unsalted	☺	Free	☺	Free of sorbitol.
Camembert cheese	☺	Free	☺	Free of sorbitol.
Cheddar cheese, natural	☺	Free	☺	Free of sorbitol.
Cheese sauce, store bought	☺	Free	☺	Free of sorbitol.
Colby Jack cheese	☺	Free	☺	Free of sorbitol.
Cottage cheese, 1% fat, lactose reduced	☺	Free	☺	Free of sorbitol.

Cold cut	SORBITOL Stand.		SORBITOL	Low sensitivity amount
Cottage cheese, uncreamed dry curd	☺	Free	☺	Free of sorbitol.
Cream cheese spread	☺	Free	☺	Free of sorbitol.
Cream cheese, whipped, flavored	☺	Free	☺	Free of sorbitol.
Cream cheese, whipped, plain	☺	Free	☺	Free of sorbitol.
Edam cheese	☺	Free	☺	Free of sorbitol.
Fleischmann's® Move Over Butter Margarine, tub	☺	Free	☺	Free of sorbitol.
Goat cheese, hard	☺	Free	☺	Free of sorbitol.
Gorgonzola cheese	☺	Free	☺	Free of sorbitol.
Gouda cheese	☺	Free	☺	Free of sorbitol.
Honey	☹	Avoid	1¼	Portion (21, 19g); 26g in total.
Hot dog, combination of meats, plain	☺	Free	☺	Free of sorbitol.
Jam or preserves	☹	Avoid	1¾	Portion (20g); 35g in total.
Jam or preserves, reduced sugar	☹	Avoid	41½	Portion (20g); 830g in total.
Jam or preserves, sugar free with aspartame	☹	Avoid	5¼	Portion (17g); 89g in total.
Jam or preserves, sugar free with saccharin	☹	Avoid	19¼	Portion (14g); 270g in total.
Jam or preserves, sugar free with sucralose	☹	Avoid	65¼	Portion (17g); 1109g in total.

Cold cut	SORBITOL Stand.		SORBITOL Low sensitivity amount	
Jam or preserves, without sugar or artificial sweetener	☹	Avoid	☹	Avoid consumption!
Kraft® Cheese Spread, Roka Blue	☺	Free	☺	Free of sorbitol.
Limburger cheese	☺	Free	☺	Free of sorbitol.
Maple syrup, pure	☺	Free	☺	Free of sorbitol.
Margarine, diet, fat free	☺	Free	☺	Free of sorbitol.
Margarine, tub, salted, sunflower oil	☺	Free	☺	Free of sorbitol.
Marmalade, sugar free with aspartame	☹	Avoid	5¼	Portion (17g); 89g in total.
Marmalade, sugar free with saccharin	☹	Avoid	16¾	Portion (16g); 268g in total.
Marmalade, sugar free with sucralose	☹	Avoid	65¼	Portion (17g); 1109g in total.
Mascarpone	☺	Free	☺	Free of sorbitol.
Mortadella	☺	Free	☺	Free of sorbitol.
Muenster cheese, natural	☺	Free	☺	Free of sorbitol.
Nutella® (filbert spread)	☹	Avoid	20¾	Portion (37g); 768g in total.
Roquefort cheese	☺	Free	☺	Free of sorbitol.
Smart Balance® Light with Flax Oil Margarine, tub	☺	Free	☺	Free of sorbitol.
Smart Balance® Margarine	☺	Free	☺	Free of sorbitol.

Cold cut	SORBITOL Stand.		SORBITOL Low sensitivity amount	
Soy Kaas Fat Free, all flavors	☹	Avoid	18½	Portion (30g); 555g in total.
Swiss cheese, natural	☺	Free	☺	Free of sorbitol.
Swiss cheese, natural, low sodium	☺	Free	☺	Free of sorbitol.
Tilsit cheese	☺	Free	☺	Free of sorbitol.

3.4.4 Dairy products

Dairy products	SORBITOL Stand.		SORBITOL Low sensitivity amount	
Almond milk, vanilla or other flavors, unsweetened	☺	Free	☺	Free of sorbitol.
Breyers® Light! Boosts Immunity Yogurt, all flavors	☹	Avoid	14¼	Piece (115g); 1639g in total.
Breyers® No Sugar Added Ice Cream, Vanilla	☹	Avoid	☹	Avoid consumption!
Breyers® YoCrunch Light Nonfat Yogurt, with granola	☹	Avoid	6½	Piece (250g); 1625g in total.
Cabot® Non Fat Yogurt, plain	☺	Free	☺	Free of sorbitol.
Cabot® Non Fat Yogurt, vanilla	☹	Avoid	13¼	Piece (150g); 1988g in total.
Chobani® Nonfat Greek Yogurt, Black Cherry	☹	Avoid	3¾	Tbsp. (15g); 56g in total.
Chobani® Nonfat Greek Yogurt, Lemon	☺	Free	☺	Free of sorbitol.
Chobani® Nonfat Greek Yogurt, Peach	☹	Avoid	4¼	Piece (250g); 1063g in total.
Chobani® Nonfat Greek Yogurt, Raspberry	☹	Avoid	20	Piece (250g); 5000g in total.
Chobani® Nonfat Greek Yogurt, Strawberry	☹	Avoid	3½	Piece (250g); 875g in total.
Chocolate pudding, store bought	☹	Avoid	25	Piece (200g); 5000g in total.
Chocolate pudding, store bought, sugar free	☹	Avoid	☹	Avoid consumption!
Cottage cheese, uncreamed dry curd	☺	Free	☺	Free of sorbitol.

Dairy products	SORBITOL Stand.		SORBITOL Low sensitivity amount	
Dannon® Activia® Light Yogurt, vanilla	Free			Free of sorbitol.
Dannon® Activia® Yogurt, plain	Free			Free of sorbitol.
Dannon® Greek Yogurt, Honey	Avoid	3¼		Piece (150g); 488g in total.
Dannon® Greek Yogurt, Plain	Free			Free of sorbitol.
Dannon® la Crème Yogurt, fruit flavors	Avoid	10¾		Piece (115g); 1236g in total.
Evaporated milk, diluted, 2% fat (reduced fat)	Free			Free of sorbitol.
Evaporated milk, diluted, skim (fat free)	Free			Free of sorbitol.
Evaporated milk, diluted, whole	Free			Free of sorbitol.
Feta cheese	Free			Free of sorbitol.
Feta cheese, fat free	Free			Free of sorbitol.
Fondue sauce	Avoid	5		Portion (53g); 265g in total.
GO Veggie!™ Rice Slices, all flavors	Free			Free of sorbitol.
Greek yogurt, plain, nonfat,	Free			Free of sorbitol.
Half and half	Free			Free of sorbitol.
Kefir	Free			Free of sorbitol.
Laughing Cow® Mini Babybel®, Cheddar	Free			Free of sorbitol.

Dairy products	SORBITOL Stand.		SORBITOL Low sensitivity amount	
Laughing Cow® Mini Babybel®, Original	☺ Free		☺	Free of sorbitol.
Licuado, mango	☹ Avoid	1		Glass (200g); 200 mL in total.
Light cream	☺ Free		☺	Free of sorbitol.
Milk, lactose reduced Lactaid®, skim (fat free)	☺ Free		☺	Free of sorbitol.
Milk, lactose reduced Lactaid®, whole	☺ Free		☺	Free of sorbitol.
Milk, lactose reduced, skim (fat free), calcium, Lactaid®	☺ Free		☺	Free of sorbitol.
Mozzarella cheese, fat free	☺ Free		☺	Free of sorbitol.
Mozzarella cheese, whole milk	☺ Free		☺	Free of sorbitol.
Oat milk	☺ Free		☺	Free of sorbitol.
Parmesan cheese, dry (grated)	☺ Free		☺	Free of sorbitol.
Parmesan cheese, dry (grated), nonfat	☺ Free		☺	Free of sorbitol.
Pudding mix, other flavors, cooked type	☺ Free		☺	Free of sorbitol.
Rice milk, plain or original, unsweetened, enriched, ready	☺ Free		☺	Free of sorbitol.
Rice pudding (arroz con leche), coconut, raisins	☹ Avoid	1 ¼		Piece (200g); 250g in total.
Rice pudding (arroz con leche), plain	☺ Free		☺	Free of sorbitol.
Rice pudding (arroz con leche), raisins	☹ Avoid	1 ¼		Piece (200g); 250g in total.

Dairy products	SORBITOL Stand.		SORBITOL Low sensitivity amount	
Ricotta cheese, part skim milk	☺ Free		☺ Free of sorbitol.	
Slim-Fast® Easy to Digest, Vanilla, ready-to-drink can	☺ Free		☺ Free of sorbitol.	
Sour cream	☺ Free		☺ Free of sorbitol.	
Soy milk, plain or original, artificial sweetener, ready	☹ Avoid		1½	Glass (200g); 300 mL in total.
Soy milk, vanilla or other flavors, sugar, fat free, ready	☹ Avoid		7	Glass (200g); 1400 mL in total.
Stonyfield® Oikos Greek Yogurt, Blueberry	☺ Free		☺ Free of sorbitol.	
Stonyfield® Oikos Greek Yogurt, Caramel	☺ Free		☺ Free of sorbitol.	
Stonyfield® Oikos Greek Yogurt, Chocolate	☺ Free		☺ Free of sorbitol.	
Stonyfield® Oikos Greek Yogurt, Strawberry	☹ Avoid		2	Piece (250g); 500g in total.
Strawberry milk, plain, prepared	☺ Free		☺ Free of sorbitol.	
Sweetened condensed milk	☺ Free		☺ Free of sorbitol.	
Sweetened condensed milk, reduced fat	☺ Free		☺ Free of sorbitol.	
Tofu, raw (not silken), cooked, low fat	☹ Avoid		¾	Portion (85g); 64g in total.
Whipped cream, aerosol	☺ Free		☺ Free of sorbitol.	
Whipped cream, aerosol, chocolate	☺ Nearly free		☺ Nearly free of sorbitol	
Whipped cream, aerosol, fat free	☺ Free		☺ Free of sorbitol.	

Dairy products	SORBITOL Stand.		SORBITOL Low sensitivity amount	
Yogurt, chocolate or coffee flavors, nonfat, aspartame	☺	Free	☺	Free of sorbitol.
Yogurt, chocolate or coffee flavors, whole milk, sucralose	☺	Free	☺	Free of sorbitol.
Yogurt, fruited, whole milk	☹	Avoid	🥄	60½ Tbsp. (15g); 908g in total.

3.4.5 Nuts and snacks

Nuts and snacks	SORBITOL Stand.		SORBITOL Low sensitivity amount
Almonds, raw	Free		Free of sorbitol.
Baby food, zwieback	Free		Free of sorbitol.
Brazil nuts, unsalted	Free		Free of sorbitol.
Caramel or sugar coated popcorn, store bought	Free		Free of sorbitol.
Cashews, raw	Free		Free of sorbitol.
Cheese cracker	Free		Free of sorbitol.
Chestnuts, roasted	Avoid	3	Portion (30g); 90g in total.
Chia seeds	Free		Free of sorbitol.
Coconut cream (liquid from grated meat)	Free		Free of sorbitol.
Coconut milk, fresh (liquid from grated meat)	Free		Free of sorbitol.
Coconut, dried, shredded or flaked, unsweetened	Free		Free of sorbitol.
Coconut, fresh	Free		Free of sorbitol.
Doritos® Tortilla Chips, Nacho Cheese	Nearly free		Nearly free of sorbitol
Filberts, raw	Avoid	8¼	Hand (30g); 248g in total.
Flax seeds, not fortified	Free		Free of sorbitol.

Nuts and snacks	SORBITOL Stand.		SORBITOL Low sensitivity amount
Ginko nuts, dried	☺ Free		☺ Free of sorbitol.
Hickorynuts	☺ Free		☺ Free of sorbitol.
Lay's® Potato Chips, Classic	☹ Avoid	79¼	Hand (21g); 1664g in total.
Lay's® Potato Chips, Salt & Vinegar	☹ Avoid	79¼	Hand (21g); 1664g in total.
Lay's® Potato Chips, Sour Cream & Onion	☹ Avoid	79¼	Hand (21g); 1664g in total.
Lay's® Stax Potato Crisps, Cheddar	☹ Avoid	79¼	Hand (21g); 1664g in total.
Lay's® Stax Potato Crisps, Hot 'n Spicy Barbecue	☺ Nearly free		☺ Nearly free of sorbitol
Macadamia nuts, raw	☺ Free		☺ Free of sorbitol.
Melba Toast®, Classic (Old London®)	☺ Nearly free		☺ Nearly free of sorbitol
Old Dutch® Crunch Curls	☺ Nearly free		☺ Nearly free of sorbitol
Peanut butter, unsalted	☺ Free		☺ Free of sorbitol.
Peanuts, dry roasted, salted	☺ Free		☺ Free of sorbitol.
Pine nuts, pignolias	☺ Free		☺ Free of sorbitol.
Pistachio nuts, raw	☺ Free		☺ Free of sorbitol.
Poore Brothers® Potato Chips, Salt & Cracked Pepper	☺ Nearly free		☺ Nearly free of sorbitol
Potato chips, salted	☹ Avoid	79¼	Hand (21g); 1664g in total.

Nuts and snacks	SORBITOL Stand.		SORBITOL Low sensitivity amount	
Potato sticks	☹ Avoid	79¼		Hand (21g); 1664g in total.
Pretzels, hard, unsalted, sticks	☺ Free			Free of sorbitol.
Pringles® Light Fat Free Potato Crisps, Barbecue	☹ Avoid	79¼		Hand (21g); 1664g in total.
Pringles® Potato Crisps, Loaded Baked Potato	☹ Avoid	79¼		Hand (21g); 1664g in total.
Pringles® Potato Crisps, Original	☺ Nearly free			Nearly free of sorbitol
Pringles® Potato Crisps, Salt & Vinegar	☹ Avoid	79¼		Hand (21g); 1664g in total.
Pumpkin or squash seeds, shelled, unsalted	☺ Free			Free of sorbitol.
Rice cake	☺ Free			Free of sorbitol.
Ritz Cracker (Nabisco®)	☺ Free			Free of sorbitol.
Sesame sticks	☺ Nearly free			Nearly free of sorbitol
Soy chips	☹ Avoid	1		Hand (21g); 21g in total.
Sunflower seeds, raw	☺ Free			Free of sorbitol.
Taco John's® nachos	☺ Nearly free			Nearly free of sorbitol
Tortilla, white, store bought, fried	☺ Free			Free of sorbitol.
Walnuts	☺ Free			Free of sorbitol.
Wise Onion Flavored Rings	☺ Nearly free			Nearly free of sorbitol

3.4.6 Sweet pastries

Sweet pastries	SORBITOL Stand.	SORBITOL Low sensitivity amount	
Almond cookies	☺ Free		☺ Free of sorbitol.
Apple cake, glazed	☹ Avoid	½	Piece (45g); 23g in total.
Apple strudel	☹ Avoid	¼	Piece (64g); 16g in total.
Archway® Ginger Snaps	☺ Free		☺ Free of sorbitol.
Archway® Oatmeal Raisin Cookies	☹ Avoid	10¼	Piece (26g); 267g in total.
Archway® Peanut Butter Cookies	☹ Avoid	10¾	Piece (34g); 366g in total.
Biscotti, chocolate, nuts	☺ Nearly free		☺ Nearly free of sorbitol
Brownie, chocolate, fat free	☺ Nearly free		☺ Nearly free of sorbitol
Butter cracker	☺ Free		☺ Free of sorbitol.
Carrot cake, glazed, homemade	☹ Avoid	8	Piece (27, 72g); 222g in total.
Cheesecake, plain or flavored, graham cracker crust, homemade	☺ Free		☺ Free of sorbitol.
Cherry pie, bottom crust only	☹ Avoid		☹ Avoid consumption!
Chips Ahoy!® Chewy Gooey Caramel Cookies (Nabisco®)	☺ Nearly free		☺ Nearly free of sorbitol
Chocolate cake, glazed, store bought	☺ Nearly free		☺ Nearly free of sorbitol

Sweet pastries	SORBITOL Stand.		SORBITOL Low sensitivity amount	
Chocolate chip cookies, store bought	☺	Nearly free	☺	Nearly free of sorbitol
Chocolate cookies, iced, store bought	☺	Nearly free	☺	Nearly free of sorbitol
Chocolate sandwich cookies, double filling	☺	Nearly free	☺	Nearly free of sorbitol
Chocolate sandwich cookies, sugar free	☹	Avoid	☹	Avoid consumption!!
Cinnamon crispas (fried flour tortilla, cinnamon, sugar)	☺	Free	☺	Free of sorbitol.
Crepe, plain	☺	Free	☺	Free of sorbitol.
Croissant, chocolate	☺	Nearly free	☺	Nearly free of sorbitol
Croissant, fruit	☹	Avoid	2	Piece (74g); 148g in total.
Danish pastry, frosted or glazed, with cheese filling	☺	Free	☺	Free of sorbitol.
Dare Breaktime Ginger Cookies	☺	Free	☺	Free of sorbitol.
Dare® Lemon Crème Cookies	☺	Free	☺	Free of sorbitol.
Doughnut, raised, glazed, coconut topping	☺	Free	☺	Free of sorbitol.
Doughnut, raised, glazed, plain	☺	Free	☺	Free of sorbitol.
Doughnut, raised, sugared	☺	Free	☺	Free of sorbitol.
EGG® bread roll	☺	Free	☺	Free of sorbitol.
Elephant ear (crispy)	☺	Free	☺	Free of sorbitol.

Sweet pastries	SORBITOL Stand.		SORBITOL Low sensitivity amount	
English muffin, whole wheat, with raisins	Avoid	2¼	Piece (66g); 149g in total.	
French toast, homemade, French bread	Free		Free of sorbitol.	
Frozen custard, chocolate or coffee flavors	Nearly free		Nearly free of sorbitol	
German chocolate cake, glazed, homemade	Nearly free		Nearly free of sorbitol	
Girl Scout® Lemonades	Free		Free of sorbitol.	
Girl Scout® Peanut Butter Patties	Nearly free		Nearly free of sorbitol	
Girl Scout® Samoas®	Avoid	¾	Piece (14.5g); 11g in total.	
Girl Scout® Shortbread®	Free		Free of sorbitol.	
Girl Scout® Thin Mints	Nearly free		Nearly free of sorbitol	
Halvah	Free		Free of sorbitol.	
Lebkuchen (German ginger bread)	Avoid	6½	Piece (32.4g); 211g in total.	
Little Debbie® Coffee Cake, Apple Streusel	Avoid	½	Piece (52g); 26g in total.	
Little Debbie® Fudge Brownies with Walnuts	Nearly free		Nearly free of sorbitol	
Long John / Bismarck, glazed, cream or custard filled, nuts	Free		Free of sorbitol.	
Molasses cookies, store bought	Free		Free of sorbitol.	
Muffins, banana	Avoid	29¼	Piece (113g); 3305g in total.	

Sweet pastries	SORBITOL Stand.		SORBITOL Low sensitivity amount	
Muffins, blueberry, store bought	☺ Free		☺	Free of sorbitol.
Muffins, carrot, homemade, with nuts	☹ Avoid	3¼		Piece (113g); 367g in total.
Muffins, oat bran or oatmeal, store bought	☺ Free		☺	Free of sorbitol.
Muffins, pumpkin, store bought	☹ Avoid	14½		Piece (113g); 1639g in total.
Murray® Sugar Free Oatmeal Cookies	☹ Avoid		☹	Avoid consumption!
Murray® Sugar Free Shortbread	☹ Avoid		☹	Avoid consumption!
Nabisco® 100 Calorie Packs, Honey Maid Cinnamon Roll	☹ Avoid	42½		Piece (13g); 553g in total.
Nilla Wafers® (Nabisco®)	☺ Free		☺	Free of sorbitol.
Nutter Butter® Cookies (Nabisco®)	☺ Free		☺	Free of sorbitol.
Oatmeal cookies, store bought	☺ Free		☺	Free of sorbitol.
Oreo® Brownie Cookies (Nabisco®)	☺ Nearly free		☺	Nearly free of sorbitol
Oreo® Cookies (Nabisco®)	☺ Nearly free		☺	Nearly free of sorbitol
Oreo® Cookies, Sugar Free (Nabisco®)	☹ Avoid		☹	Avoid consumption!!
Pancake, buckwheat, from mix, add water only	☹ Avoid	3¾		Piece (44g); 165g in total.
Pancake, whole wheat, homemade	☺ Free		☺	Free of sorbitol.
Peach pie, bottom crust only	☹ Avoid	1		Piece (122g); 122g in total.

Sweet pastries	SORBITOL Stand.		SORBITOL Low sensitivity amount	
Pepperidge Farm® Sweet & Simple, Soft Sugar Cookies	Free			Free of sorbitol.
Pepperidge Farm® Turnover, Apple	Avoid	¼		Piece (89g); 22g in total.
Pillsbury® Big White Chunk Macadamia Nut Cookies	Free			Free of sorbitol.
Pillsbury® Cinnamon Roll with Icing, all flavors	Free			Free of sorbitol.
Popcorn, store bought (prepopped), "buttered"	Free			Free of sorbitol.
Rhubarb pie, bottom crust only	Free			Free of sorbitol.
Sandwich cookies, vanilla	Free			Free of sorbitol.
Sticky bun	Free			Free of sorbitol.
Strawberry pie, bottom crust only	Avoid	¾		Piece (122g); 92g in total.
Sugar cookies, iced, store bought	Free			Free of sorbitol.
Sweet potato bread	Free			Free of sorbitol.
Tiramisu	Free			Free of sorbitol.
Twix®	Free			Free of sorbitol.
Waffles, bran	Free			Free of sorbitol.
Waffles, whole wheat, from mix, add milk, fat and egg	Free			Free of sorbitol.
Windmill cookies	Free			Free of sorbitol.

3.4.7 Sweets

Sweets	SORBITOL Stand.		SORBITOL Low sensitivity amount	
3 Musketeers®	Free		Free of sorbitol.	
After Eight® Thin Chocolate Mints	Free		Free of sorbitol.	
Almond paste (Marzipan)	Avoid	20½	Portion (28.38g); 582g in total.	
Almonds, honey roasted	Avoid	5½	Hand (30g); 165g in total.	
Breath mint, regular	Free		Free of sorbitol.	
Breath mint, sugar free	Avoid		Avoid consumption!!	
Brown sugar	Free		Free of sorbitol.	
Buttermels® (Switzer's®)	Free		Free of sorbitol.	
Candy necklace	Free		Free of sorbitol.	
Chewing gum	Free		Free of sorbitol.	
Chewing gum, sugar free	Avoid		Avoid consumption!	
Chocolate truffles	Free		Free of sorbitol.	
Classic Fruit Chocolates (Liberty Orchards®)	Avoid	31½	Piece (15g); 473g in total.	
Coconut Bars, nuts	Free		Free of sorbitol.	
Dark chocolate Bar 45%-59% cacao	Avoid	8	135g Bar (125g); 1000g in total.	

Sweets	SORBITOL Stand.		SORBITOL Low sensitivity amount	
Dark chocolate Bar 60%-69% cacao	☹ Avoid	6½		135g Bar (125g); 813g in total.
Dark chocolate Bar 70%-85% cacao	☹ Avoid	5		135g Bar (125g); 625g in total.
Dark chocolate Bar, sugar free	☹ Avoid		☹	Avoid consumption!!
Dark Fruit Chocolates (Liberty Orchards®)	☹ Avoid	31½		Piece (15g); 473g in total.
Dark Fruit Chocolates, Sugar Free (Liberty Orchards®)	☹ Avoid		☹	Avoid consumption!!
Fifty 50® Sugar Free Low Glycemic Butterscotch Hard Candy	☹ Avoid		☹	Avoid consumption!!
French Burnt Peanuts	☺ Free		☺	Free of sorbitol.
Gelatin (jello) powder, flavored, sugar free	☺ Free		☺	Free of sorbitol.
Gelatin (jello) powder, plain	☺ Free		☺	Free of sorbitol.
Gum drops	☺ Free		☺	Free of sorbitol.
Gum drops, sugar free	☹ Avoid		☹	Avoid consumption!!
Gummi bears	☺ Nearly free		☺	Nearly free of sorbitol
Gummi bears, sugar free	☹ Avoid		☹	Avoid consumption!!
Gummi dinosaurs	☺ Nearly free		☺	Nearly free of sorbitol
Gummi dinosaurs, sugar free	☹ Avoid		☹	Avoid consumption!!
Gummi worms	☺ Nearly free		☺	Nearly free of sorbitol

Sweets	SORBITOL Stand.		SORBITOL Low sensitivity amount	
Gummi worms, sugar free		Avoid		Avoid consumption!!
Hard candy		Free		Free of sorbitol.
Hard candy, sugar free		Avoid		Avoid consumption!!
Hershey's® Caramel Filled Chocolates Sugar Free		Avoid		Avoid consumption!!
Hershey's® Milk Chocolate Bar		Free		Free of sorbitol.
Jelly beans®		Free		Free of sorbitol.
Jelly beans®, sugar free		Avoid		Avoid consumption!!
Jujyfruits®		Free		Free of sorbitol.
Kashi® Layered Granola Bar, Pumpkin Pecan		Avoid	25	Piece (40g); 1000g in total.
Kit Kat®		Nearly free		Nearly free of sorbitol
Kit Kat® White		Free		Free of sorbitol.
Licorice		Free		Free of sorbitol.
Little Debbie® Nutty Bars		Nearly free		Nearly free of sorbitol
M & M's® Peanut		Free		Free of sorbitol.
Mamba® Fruit Chews		Avoid		Avoid consumption!!
Mamba® Sour Fruit Chews		Avoid		Avoid consumption!!

Sweets	SORBITOL Stand.		SORBITOL Low sensitivity amount	
Marshmallow	Free			Free of sorbitol.
Mentos®	Free			Free of sorbitol.
Milk chocolate Bar, cereal	Avoid	40		135g Bar (125g); 5000g in total.
Milk chocolate Bar, cereal, sugar free	Avoid			Avoid consumption!!
Milk chocolate Bar, sugar free	Avoid			Avoid consumption!!
Milk Chocolate covered raisins	Avoid	3¼		Hand (30g); 98g in total.
Milk Maid® Caramels (Brach's®)	Free			Free of sorbitol.
Molasses, dark	Free			Free of sorbitol.
Nestle® Nesquik®, chocolate flavors, unprepared dry	Avoid	5½		Glass (200g); 1100 mL in total.
Nougat	Free			Free of sorbitol.
Pecan praline	Free			Free of sorbitol.
Riesen®	Avoid			Avoid consumption!!
Smarties®	Free			Free of sorbitol.
Snickers®	Free			Free of sorbitol.
Snickers®, Almond	Free			Free of sorbitol.
Splenda®	Free			Free of sorbitol.

Sweets	SORBITOL Stand.		SORBITOL Low sensitivity amount
Starburst®, Original	Avoid	30¼	Piece (5g); 151g in total.
Suckers®, sugar free	Avoid		Avoid consumption!!
Sugar, white granulated	Free		Free of sorbitol.
Taffy	Free		Free of sorbitol.
Tic Tacs®	Free		Free of sorbitol.
Toblerone® Swiss Dark Chocolate with Honey & Almond Nougat	Avoid	40	Piece (25g); 1000g in total.
Toblerone® Swiss Milk Chocolate with Honey & Almond Nougat	Free		Free of sorbitol.
Toblerone® Swiss White Confection with Honey & Almond Nougat	Free		Free of sorbitol.
Toffee	Free		Free of sorbitol.
Toffifay®	Avoid		Avoid consumption!
Tootsie Pops®	Free		Free of sorbitol.
Werther's® Original Caramel Coffee Hard Candies	Free		Free of sorbitol.
White chocolate Bar	Free		Free of sorbitol.
Wild 'n Fruity Gummi Bears (Brach's®)	Nearly free		Nearly free of sorbitol
Zsweet®	Avoid		Avoid consumption!!

3.5 Warm dishes

3.5.1 Meals

Meals	SORBITOL Stand.		SORBITOL Low sensitivity amount	
Arby's® macaroni and cheese	Free			Free of sorbitol.
Asian noodle bowl, vegetables only	Avoid	10		Portion (200g); 2000g in total.
Baby food, Gerber Graduates® Organic Pasta Pick-Ups Three Cheese Ravioli	Free			Free of sorbitol.
Beef with noodles soup, condensed	Avoid	4¼		Portion (126g); 536g in total.
Boston Market® macaroni and cheese	Free			Free of sorbitol.
Butternut squash soup	Avoid	2½		Portion (245g); 613g in total.
Calzone, cheese	Avoid	2¾		Piece (168g); 462g in total.
Casserole (hot dish), pasta with turkey, gravy base, vegeexcept dark green, & cheese	Avoid	1¼		Portion (228g); 285g in total.
Casserole (hot dish), rice with beef, tomato base, vegetables except dark green, & cheese	Avoid	¼		Portion (244g); 61g in total.
Chicken and dumplings soup, condensed	Avoid	2¼		Portion (126g); 284g in total.
Chicken noodle soup with vegetables, ready-to-serve can	Avoid	1		Portion (245g); 245g in total.
Chicken wonton soup, prepared from condensed can	Avoid	40¾		Portion (245g); 9984g in total.
Chili with beans, beef, canned	Avoid	55½		Tbsp. (15g); 833g in total.

Meals	SORBITOL Stand.		SORBITOL Low sensitivity amount	
Chop suey, chicken, no noodles	☹	Avoid	¼	Portion (166g); 42g in total.
Chop suey, tofu, no noodles	☹	Avoid	¼	Portion (166g); 42g in total.
Cream of asparagus soup, prepared from condensed can	☺	Nearly free	☺	Nearly free of sorbitol
Cream of broccoli soup, condensed	☹	Avoid	19¾	Portion (126g); 2489g in total.
Cream of celery soup, homemade	☹	Avoid	¼	Portion (245g); 61g in total.
Cream of chicken soup, condensed	☹	Avoid	26¼	Portion (126g); 3308g in total.
Cream of mushroom soup, prepared from condensed can	☹	Avoid	¼	Portion (245g); 61g in total.
Cream of potato soup mix, dry	☹	Avoid	3	Portion (23g); 69g in total.
Cream of spinach soup mix, dry	☹	Avoid	18¼	Portion (17g); 310g in total.
Dairy Queen® Foot Long Hot Dog	☹	Avoid	8¼	Piece (199g); 1642g in total.
Fettuccini Alfredo®, no meat, vegetables except dark green	☹	Avoid	¼	Portion (200g); 50g in total.
Fettuccini Alfredo®, no meat, carrots / dark green veggies	☺	Free	☺	Free of sorbitol.
Fruit sauce, jelly-based	☹	Avoid	¾	Portion (40g); 30g in total.
German style potato salad, bacon and vinegar dressing	☹	Avoid	4¾	Portion (140g); 665g in total.
Green pea soup, prepared from condensed can	☹	Avoid	20	Tbsp. (15g); 300g in total.
Hardee's® Loaded Omelet Biscuit	☺	Free	☺	Free of sorbitol.

Meals	SORBITOL Stand.		SORBITOL Low sensitivity amount	
Lasagna, homemade, beef	☹	Avoid	1	Portion (140g); 140g in total.
Lasagna, homemade, cheese, no vegetables	☹	Avoid	¾	Portion (140g); 105g in total.
Lasagna, homemade, spinach, no meat	☹	Avoid	½	Portion (140g); 70g in total.
Lentil soup, condensed	☹	Avoid	1	Portion (126g); 126g in total.
Lyonnaise (potatoes and onions)	☹	Avoid	15¾	Portion (70g); 1103g in total.
Macaroni or pasta salad, with meat, egg, mayo dressing	☹	Avoid	1¼	Portion (140g); 175g in total.
Meat ravioli, with tomato sauce	☹	Avoid	½	Portion (250g); 125g in total.
Minestrone soup, condensed	☹	Avoid	¾	Portion (126g); 95g in total.
Minestrone soup, homemade	☹	Avoid	1	Portion (245g); 245g in total.
Noodle soup mix, dry	☺	Free	☺	Free of sorbitol.
Omelet, made with bacon	☺	Free	☺	Free of sorbitol.
Omelet, made with sausage, potatoes, onions, cheese	☹	Avoid	6¾	Portion (110g); 743g in total.
Pad Thai, without meat	☹	Avoid	3¾	Portion (140g); 525g in total.
Paella	☹	Avoid	2¼	Portion (240g); 540g in total.
Panda Express® Orange Chicken	☹	Avoid	23¾	Portion (140g); 3325g in total.
Pasta salad with vegetables, Italian dressing	☹	Avoid	1½	Portion (140g); 210g in total.

Meals	SORBITOL Stand.		SORBITOL Low sensitivity amount	
Pho soup (Vietnamese noodle soup)	Avoid	6¾	Portion (245g); 1654g in total.
Pizza Hut® cheese bread stick	Free		Free of sorbitol.
Pizza Hut® Pepperoni Lover's pizza, stuffed crust	Avoid	1	Portion (140g); 140g in total.
Pizza Hut® Personal Pan, supreme	Avoid	¼	Piece (256g); 64g in total.
Pizza, homemade or restaurant, cheese, thin crust	Avoid	¾	Piece (209g); 157g in total.
Potato salad, with egg, mayo dressing	Avoid	2	Portion (140g); 280g in total.
Potato soup with broccoli and cheese	Avoid	13½	Portion (245g); 3308g in total.
Ratatouille	Avoid	1¼	Portion (110g); 138g in total.
Red beans and rice soup mix, dry	Avoid	¼	Portion (51.03g); 13g in total.
Scrambled egg, made with bacon	Free		Free of sorbitol.
Sesame chicken	Avoid	3¾	Portion (252g); 945g in total.
Soup base	Avoid	74	Tbsp. (15g); 1110g in total.
Spaghetti, with carbonara sauce	Avoid	6	Portion (201g); 1206g in total.
Spinach ravioli, with tomato sauce	Avoid	½	Portion (250g); 125g in total.
Spring roll	Avoid	2¾	Portion (140g); 385g in total.
Squash or pumpkin ravioli, with cream sauce	Avoid	40	Portion (250g); 10000g in total.

Meals	SORBITOL Stand.		SORBITOL Low sensitivity amount	
Stewed green peas with sofrito	Avoid	5½		Tbsp. (15g); 83g in total.
Sushi, with fish	Avoid	2½		Portion (140g); 350g in total.
Sushi, with fish and vegetables in seaweed	Avoid	2		Portion (140g); 280g in total.
Sushi, with vegetables in seaweed	Avoid	1½		Portion (140g); 210g in total.
Swedish Meatballs	Avoid	71¼		Portion (140g); 9975g in total.
Sweet and sour chicken	Nearly free			Nearly free of sorbitol
Taco Bell® 7-Layer Burrito	Avoid	5¾		Portion (140g); 805g in total.
Taco Bell® Crunchwrap Supreme	Avoid	5		Piece (245g); 1225g in total.
Taco Bell® Mexican Pizza	Avoid	1		Piece (213g); 213g in total.
Taco Bell® Nachos Supreme	Avoid	7¾		Portion (140g); 1085g in total.
Taco, soft corn shell, with beans, cheese	Avoid	4¼		Portion (140g); 595g in total.
Tomato relish	Avoid	5¼		Portion (15g); 79g in total.
Tomato soup mix, dry	Avoid	2		Portion (34.66g); 69g in total.
Vegetable soup, condensed	Avoid	1		Portion (126g); 126g in total.
Vichyssoise	Avoid	1¼		Portion (245g); 306g in total.
White bean stew with sofrito	Nearly free			Nearly free of sorbitol

3.5.2 Meat and fish

Meat and fish	SORBITOL Stand.		SORBITOL Low sensitivity amount	
Arby's® Chicken Cordon Bleu Sandwich, crispy	☺	Free	☺	Free of sorbitol.
Beef bacon (kosher)	☺	Free	☺	Free of sorbitol.
Beef steak, chuck, visible fat eaten	☺	Free	☺	Free of sorbitol.
Bockwurst	☺	Free	☺	Free of sorbitol.
Boston Market® 1/4 white rotisserie chicken, with skin	☺	Free	☺	Free of sorbitol.
Boston Market® roasted turkey breast	☺	Free	☺	Free of sorbitol.
Bratwurst	☺	Free	☺	Free of sorbitol.
Bratwurst, beef	☺	Free	☺	Free of sorbitol.
Bratwurst, light (reduced fat)	☺	Free	☺	Free of sorbitol.
Bratwurst, made with beer	☺	Nearly free	☺	Nearly free of sorbitol
Bratwurst, made with beer, cheese-filled	☺	Nearly free	☺	Nearly free of sorbitol
Bratwurst, turkey	☺	Free	☺	Free of sorbitol.
Braunschweiger	☺	Free	☺	Free of sorbitol.
Caviar	☺	Free	☺	Free of sorbitol.
Chicken fricassee with gravy, American style	☺	Free	☺	Free of sorbitol.

Meat and fish	SORBITOL Stand.		SORBITOL Low sensitivity amount	
Clams, stuffed with mushroom, onions, and bread	☹	Avoid	½ 🥄	Portion (140g); 70g in total.
Fish croquette	☺	Nearly free	☺	Nearly free of sorbitol
Fish sticks, patties, or nuggets, breaded, regular	☺	Free	☺	Free of sorbitol.
Fish with breading	☺	Free	☺	Free of sorbitol.
Gorton's® Battered Fish Fillets - Lemon Pepper	☺	Free	☺	Free of sorbitol.
Gorton's® Popcorn Shrimp, Original	☺	Free	☺	Free of sorbitol.
Goulash, with beef, noodles or macaroni, tomato base	☹	Avoid	4 🥄	Tbsp. (15g); 60g in total.
Herring, pickled	☺	Free	☺	Free of sorbitol.
Herring, pickled	☺	Free	☺	Free of sorbitol.
Liver pudding	☺	Free	☺	Free of sorbitol.
Mrs. Paul's® Calamari Rings	☺	Free	☺	Free of sorbitol.
Pickled beef	☺	Free	☺	Free of sorbitol.
Pork cutlet (sirloin cutlet), visible fat eaten	☺	Free	☺	Free of sorbitol.
Ribs, beef, spare, visible fat eaten	☺	Free	☺	Free of sorbitol.
Salami, beer or beerwurst, beef	☺	Free	☺	Free of sorbitol.
Salmon, red (sockeye), smoked	☺	Free	☺	Free of sorbitol.

Meat and fish	SORBITOL Stand.		SORBITOL Low sensitivity amount	
Sauerbraten	☺	Free	☺	Free of sorbitol.
Scallops	☺	Free	☺	Free of sorbitol.
Sea Pak® Seasoned Shrimp, Roasted Garlic	☺	Free	☺	Free of sorbitol.
Sea Pak® Shrimp Scampi in Italian Parmesan Sauce	☺	Free	☺	Free of sorbitol.
Spiced ham loaf (e.g. Spam), canned	☺	Free	☺	Free of sorbitol.
Tuna, canned, light, oil pack, not drained	☺	Free	☺	Free of sorbitol.
Venison or deer, stewed	☺	Free	☺	Free of sorbitol.

3.5.3 Side dishes

Side dishes	SORBITOL Stand.		SORBITOL Low sensitivity amount	
Au gratin potato, prepared from fresh	Avoid	7¾	Portion (140g); 1085g in total.	
Basmati rice, cooked in unsalted water	Free		Free of sorbitol.	
Boston Market® sweet corn	Avoid	4	Portion (85g); 340g in total.	
Bulgur, home cooked	Free		Free of sorbitol.	
Cheese gnocchi	Free		Free of sorbitol.	
Cornbread, from mix	Nearly free		Nearly free of sorbitol	
Cornbread, homemade	Free		Free of sorbitol.	
Couscous, cooked	Free		Free of sorbitol.	
Falafel	Avoid	1¾	Portion (55g); 96g in total.	
Fettuccini noodles, whole wheat, cooked	Free		Free of sorbitol.	
Garbanzo beans (chickpeas), canned, drained	Avoid	1	Portion (90g); 90g in total.	
Green peas, raw	Avoid	3½	Tbsp. (15g); 53g in total.	
Kidney beans, cooked from dried	Free		Free of sorbitol.	
Lentils, cooked from dried	Free		Free of sorbitol.	
Plain dumplings for stew, biscuit type	Free		Free of sorbitol.	

Side dishes	SORBITOL Stand.		SORBITOL Low sensitivity amount	
Polenta	☹ Avoid	20¾		Portion (240g); 4980g in total.
Potato dumpling (Kartoffelkloesse)	☹ Avoid	35½		Portion (140g); 4970g in total.
Potato gnocchi	☺ Free			Free of sorbitol.
Potato pancakes	☹ Avoid	12¾		Portion (70g); 893g in total.
Potato, boiled, with skin	☹ Avoid	45¼		Portion (110g); 4978g in total.
Potato, boiled, without skin	☹ Avoid	45¼		Portion (110g); 4978g in total.
Quinoa, cooked	☺ Free			Free of sorbitol.
Rice noodles, fried	☺ Free			Free of sorbitol.
Snow peas (edible pea pods), cooked from fresh	☺ Free			Free of sorbitol.
Spaetzle (spatzen)	☺ Free			Free of sorbitol.

3.6 Fast food chains

3.6.1 Burger King®

Burger King®	SORBITOL Stand.	SORBITOL Low sensitivity amount	
Bacon EGG® and Cheese BK Muffin®	☺ Free	☺	Free of sorbitol.
Barbecue sauce	☹ Avoid	2¼	Portion (31g); 70g in total.
BBQ roasted jalapeno sauce	☹ Avoid	2¾	Portion (31g); 85g in total.
BK Big Fish®	☹ Avoid	21¾	Piece (228g); 4959g in total.
BK Fresh Apple Slices	☹ Avoid	☹	Avoid consumption!
BLT Salad® with TenderCrisp chicken (no dressing or croutons)	☹ Avoid	3	Portion (140g); 420g in total.
Caesar Salad (no dressing or croutons)	☹ Avoid	4¼	Portion (100g); 425g in total.
Cheeseburger	☹ Avoid	3¼	Piece (121g); 393g in total.
French fries	☹ Avoid	35½	Portion (70g); 2485g in total.
Hamburger	☹ Avoid	3¼	Piece (109g); 354g in total.
Ken's® Apple Cider Vinaigrette salad dressing	☺ Free	☺	Free of sorbitol.
Onion rings	☹ Avoid	¾	Portion (70g); 53g in total.
Original Chicken Crisp® Sandwich	☹ Avoid	67	Piece (149g); 9983g in total.

Burger King®	SORBITOL Stand.		SORBITOL Low sensitivity amount	
Pancakes and syrup		Free		Free of sorbitol.
Picante taco sauce		Avoid	2¾	Portion (35g); 96g in total.
Ranch Crispy Chicken Wrap		Avoid	36¼	Piece (137g); 4966g in total.
Shake, chocolate		Free		Free of sorbitol.
Shake, strawberry		Avoid	3¼	Portion (229g); 744g in total.
Shake, vanilla or other		Free		Free of sorbitol.
Sundaes®, caramel		Free		Free of sorbitol.
Sundaes®, chocolate fudge		Free		Free of sorbitol.
Sundaes®, mini M & M®		Free		Free of sorbitol.
Sundaes®, Oreo®		Avoid	49	Portion (204g); 9996g in total.
Sundaes®, strawberry		Avoid	2½	Portion (141g); 353g in total.
Sweet and sour sauce		Avoid	41½	Portion (30g); 1245g in total.
TenderCrisp® Chicken Sandwich		Avoid	2½	Piece (264g); 660g in total.
Whopper® with cheese		Avoid	1	Piece (315g); 315g in total.
Zesty onion ring sauce		Avoid	64½	Portion (31g); 2000g in total.

3.6.2 KFC®

KFC®	SORBITOL Stand.		SORBITOL Low sensitivity amount	
Caesar salad dressing	☺	Free	☺	Free of sorbitol.
Chicken breast, spicy crispy	☺	Free	☺	Free of sorbitol.
Chicken Littles with sauce	☹	Avoid	33	Piece (101g); 3333g in total.
Cole slaw	☹	Avoid	2¾	Portion (100g); 275g in total.
Creamy buffalo sauce	☺	Free	☺	Free of sorbitol.
Crispy Chicken Caesar Salad	☹	Avoid	17¾	Portion (140g); 2485g in total.
Crispy Twister without sauce	☹	Avoid	2	Piece (218g); 436g in total.
Crispy Twister® with sauce	☹	Avoid	2	Piece (240g); 480g in total.
Extra Crispy Tenders	☺	Free	☺	Free of sorbitol.
Honey BBQ sauce	☹	Avoid	2¼	Portion (31g); 70g in total.
Hot wings	☺	Free	☺	Free of sorbitol.
House side salad	☹	Avoid	4	Portion (100g); 400g in total.
Mashed potatoes with gravy	☹	Avoid	35½	Portion (140g); 4970g in total.
Sweet and sour sauce	☹	Avoid	37	Portion (30g); 1110g in total.
Sweet corn	☹	Avoid	2½	Piece (95g); 238g in total.

3.6.3 McDonald's®

McDonald's®	SORBITOL Stand.		SORBITOL Low sensitivity amount
McDonald's® apple Slices	Avoid	¼	Piece (34g); 9g in total.
McDonald's® Barbecue sauce	Avoid	1¾	Portion (31g); 54g in total.
McDonald's® Big Mac®	Avoid	6½	Piece (215g); 1398g in total.
McDonald's® caramel sundae®	Free		Free of sorbitol.
McDonald's® Cheeseburger	Avoid	5	Piece (114g); 570g in total.
McDonald's® Chicken McNuggets®	Free		Free of sorbitol.
McDonald's® chocolate chip cookies	Nearly free		Nearly free of sorbitol
McDonald's® chocolate milk	Free		Free of sorbitol.
McDonald's® Crispy Chicken Snack Wrap with ranch sauce	Avoid	84½	Piece (118g); 9971g in total.
McDonald's® Double Cheeseburger	Avoid	4¼	Piece (165g); 701g in total.
McDonald's® Filet-O-Fish®	Avoid	70¼	Piece (142g); 9976g in total.
McDonald's® French fries	Avoid	35½	Portion (70g); 2485g in total.
McDonald's® Hamburger	Avoid	5	Piece (100g); 500g in total.
McDonald's® hot fudge sundae®	Avoid	55¾	Portion (179g); 9979g in total.
McDonald's® hot mustard sauce	Free		Free of sorbitol.

McDonald's®	SORBITOL Stand.	SORBITOL Low sensitivity amount	
McDonald's® M & M McFlurry®	☺ Free	☺	Free of sorbitol.
McDonald's® McCafe shakes, chocolate flavors	☹ Avoid	15¾	Portion (210g); 3308g in total.
McDonald's® McCafe shakes, vanilla or other flavors	☹ Avoid	12	Portion (206g); 2472g in total.
McDonald's® McChicken®	☹ Avoid	69¾	Piece (143g); 9974g in total.
McDonald's® McDouble®	☹ Avoid	4¼	Piece (151g); 642g in total.
McDonald's® McRib®	☹ Avoid	1¾	Piece (208g); 364g in total.
McDonald's® Newman's Own® Creamy Caesar salad dressing	☹ Avoid	7¼	Portion (30g); 218g in total.
McDonald's® Newman's Own® Low Fat Balsamic Vinaigrette salad dressing	☺ Free	☺	Free of sorbitol.
McDonald's® orange juice	☹ Avoid	¼	Glass (200g); 50 mL in total.
McDonald's® Quarter Pounder	☹ Avoid	2½	Piece (173g); 433g in total.
McDonald's® Sausage & EGG® McMuffin®	☺ Free	☺	Free of sorbitol.
McDonald's® side salad	☹ Avoid	2½	Portion (100g); 250g in total.
McDonald's® smoothies, all flavors	☹ Avoid	1¼	Glass (200g); 250 mL in total.
McDonald's® Southwestern chipotle Barbecue sauce	☹ Avoid	2¾	Portion (31g); 85g in total.
McDonald's® sweet and sour sauce	☹ Avoid	41½	Portion (30g); 1245g in total.

3.6.4 Subway®

Subway®	SORBITOL Stand.		SORBITOL Low sensitivity amount
9-grain Wheat bread	Free		Free of sorbitol.
American cheese	Free		Free of sorbitol.
Bacon	Free		Free of sorbitol.
Cheddar cheese	Free		Free of sorbitol.
Chipotle southwest salad dressing	Free		Free of sorbitol.
Chocolate chip cookie	Nearly free		Nearly free of sorbitol
Chocolate chunk cookie	Nearly free		Nearly free of sorbitol
Ham Sandwich with Veggies, no mayo	Avoid	1 ¼	Piece (219g); 274g in total.
Honey mustard salad dressing	Free		Free of sorbitol.
Honey Oat bread	Avoid	6 ½	Piece (89g); 579g in total.
Italian BMT® Sandwich with Veggies, no mayo	Avoid	1 ¼	Piece (226g); 283g in total.
M & M® cookie	Nearly free		Nearly free of sorbitol
Mustard	Free		Free of sorbitol.
Oven Roasted Chicken Sandwich with Veggies, no mayo	Avoid	1 ¼	Piece (233g); 291g in total.
Parmesan Oregano bread	Free		Free of sorbitol.

Subway®	SORBITOL Stand.		SORBITOL Low sensitivity amount	
Ranch salad dressing	☺	Nearly free		Nearly free of sorbitol
Roast Beef Sandwich with Veggies, no mayo	☹	Avoid	1¼	Piece (233g); 291g in total.
Spicy Italian Sandwich with Veggies, no meat	☹	Avoid	1¼	Piece (222g); 278g in total.
Steak & Cheese Sandwich with Veggies, no mayo	☹	Avoid	1¼	Piece (245g); 306g in total.
Sweet Onion Chicken Teriyaki Sandwich with Veggies, no mayo	☹	Avoid	1¼	Piece (276g); 345g in total.
Sweet onion salad dressing	☹	Avoid	55½	Portion (30g); 1665g in total.
Tuna Sandwich with Veggies, no mayo	☹	Avoid	1¼	Piece (233g); 291g in total.
Turkey Breast & Ham Sandwich with Veggies, no mayo	☹	Avoid	1¼	Piece (219g); 274g in total.
Turkey Breast Sandwich with Veggies, no mayo	☹	Avoid	1¼	Piece (219g); 274g in total.
Veggie Delite Salad, no dressing	☹	Avoid	2¼	Portion (100g); 225g in total.
Veggie Delite Sandwich, no mayo	☹	Avoid	1½	Piece (162g); 243g in total.
Vinegar	☹	Avoid	20¼	Portion (14.94g); 303g in total.
White chip macadamia nut cookie	☺	Free		Free of sorbitol.
Wrap bread	☺	Free		Free of sorbitol.

3.6.5 Taco Bell®

Taco Bell®	SORBITOL Stand.		SORBITOL Low sensitivity amount	
Chalupas Supreme® with beef, beans, cheese	Avoid	1¾		Portion (140g); 245g in total.
Taco Bell® Beef Enchirito	Avoid	2¼		Portion (140g); 315g in total.
Taco Bell® Caramel Apple Empanada	Avoid			Avoid consumption!
Taco Bell® Cheesy Fiesta Potatos	Avoid	35½		Portion (140g); 4970g in total.
Taco Bell® cheesy gordita crunch	Free			Free of sorbitol.
Taco Bell® Cinnamon Twists	Free			Free of sorbitol.
Taco Bell® Combo Burrito	Avoid	4¾		Portion (140g); 665g in total.
Taco Bell® Double Decker Taco Supreme®, beef	Avoid	7		Portion (140g); 980g in total.
Taco Bell® Pintos 'n Cheese	Avoid	3¼		Portion (130g); 423g in total.

3.6.6 Wendy's®

Wendy's®	SORBITOL Stand.	SORBITOL Low sensitivity amount	
Strawberry Shake	Avoid	3¼	Glass (200g); 650 mL in total.
Wendys' chili cheese fries	Avoid	2¾	Portion (140g); 385g in total.
Wendy's® Baconator®	Avoid	23¾	Portion (140g); 3325g in total.
Wendy's® Baked Potato, with sour cream and chives	Avoid	35½	Portion (140g); 4970g in total.
Wendy's® Caesar side salad	Avoid	4¼	Portion (100g); 425g in total.
Wendy's® Chicken Nuggets	Free		Free of sorbitol.
Wendy's® French fries	Avoid	35½	Portion (70g); 2485g in total.
Wendy's® Frosty Float®	Free		Free of sorbitol.
Wendy's® Jr. Bacon Cheeseburger	Avoid	3¾	Portion (140g); 525g in total.
Wendy's® Jr. Cheeseburger Deluxe	Avoid	2½	Portion (140g); 350g in total.
Wendy's® side salad	Avoid	2¾	Portion (100g); 275g in total.
Wendy's® Spicy Chicken Go Wrap	Avoid	71¼	Portion (140g); 9975g in total.
Wendy's® Spicy Chicken Sandwich	Avoid	4¾	Portion (140g); 665g in total.

3.7 Fruits and vegetables

3.7.1 Fruit

Fruit	SORBITOL Stand.		SORBITOL Low sensitivity amount
Apple, fresh, with skin	Avoid		Avoid consumption!
Applesauce, canned, sweetened	Avoid	¾	Tbsp. (15g); 11g in total.
Applesauce, canned, unsweetened	Avoid	1	Tbsp. (15g); 15g in total.
Apricot, dried, cooked, sweetened	Avoid	1¼	Piece (20g); 25g in total.
Apricot, dried, uncooked	Avoid	¼	Piece (20g); 5g in total.
Apricot, fresh	Avoid	¾	Piece (35g); 26g in total.
Banana, chips	Avoid	12½	Portion (40g); 500g in total.
Banana, fresh	Avoid	9¼	Piece (118g); 1092g in total.
Blackberries, fresh	Free		Free of sorbitol.
Blueberries, fresh	Free		Free of sorbitol.
Boysenberries, fresh	Free		Free of sorbitol.
Cantaloupe, fresh	Avoid	14¼	Portion (140g); 1995g in total.
Carambola (starfruit), fresh	Avoid	1¼	Piece (91g); 114g in total.
Clementine, fresh	Free		Free of sorbitol.

Fruit	SORBITOL Stand.		SORBITOL Low sensitivity amount	
Cranberries, dried (Craisins®)	☹	Avoid	41½	Portion (40g); 1660g in total.
Cranberries, fresh	☹	Avoid	45¼	Portion (55g); 2489g in total.
Currants, fresh, black	☺	Free	☺	Free of sorbitol.
Currants, fresh, red and white	☺	Free	☺	Free of sorbitol.
Dates	☺	Free	☺	Free of sorbitol.
Elderberries, fresh	☺	Free	☺	Free of sorbitol.
Figs, dried, cooked, sweetened	☺	Free	☺	Free of sorbitol.
Figs, fresh	☺	Free	☺	Free of sorbitol.
Gooseberries, fresh	☺	Free	☺	Free of sorbitol.
Grapefruit, fresh, pink or red	☺	Free	☺	Free of sorbitol.
Grapes, fresh	☹	Avoid	½	Portion (140g); 70g in total.
Guava (guayaba), fresh, common	☹	Avoid	½	Piece (250g); 125g in total.
Honeydew	☺	Free	☺	Free of sorbitol.
Jackfruit, fresh	☹	Avoid	½	Tbsp. (15g); 8g in total.
Kiwi fruit, gold	☺	Free	☺	Free of sorbitol.
Kiwi fruit, green	☺	Free	☺	Free of sorbitol.

Fruit	SORBITOL Stand.		SORBITOL Low sensitivity amount	
Lemon, fresh	😊 Free		😊 Free of sorbitol.	
Lime, fresh	😊 Free		😊 Free of sorbitol.	
Loganberries, fresh	😊 Free		😊 Free of sorbitol.	
Lowbush cranberries (lingonberries)	☹ Avoid	35½	Portion (140g); 4970g in total.	
Lychees (litchis), fresh	😊 Free		😊 Free of sorbitol.	
Lycium (wolf or goji berries)	😊 Free		😊 Free of sorbitol.	
Mandarin orange, fresh	😊 Free		😊 Free of sorbitol.	
Mango, fresh	☹ Avoid	4	Tbsp. (15g); 60g in total.	
Mangosteen, fresh	😊 Free		😊 Free of sorbitol.	
Mulberries	😊 Free		😊 Free of sorbitol.	
Muskmelon	😊 Free		😊 Free of sorbitol.	
Nectarine, fresh	☹ Avoid	1	Tbsp. (15g); 15g in total.	
Orange, fresh	😊 Free		😊 Free of sorbitol.	
Papaya, fresh	😊 Free		😊 Free of sorbitol.	
Passion fruit (maracuya), fresh	😊 Free		😊 Free of sorbitol.	
Peach, fresh	☹ Avoid	¼	Portion (140g); 35g in total.	

Fruit	SORBITOL Stand.		SORBITOL Low sensitivity amount	
Pear, fresh	Avoid	¼		Tbsp. (15g); 4g in total.
Persimmon, fresh	Free			Free of sorbitol.
Pineapple, dried	Avoid	½		Portion (40g); 20g in total.
Pineapple, fresh	Avoid	¾		Portion (140g); 105g in total.
Plantains, green, boiled	Free			Free of sorbitol.
Plum, fresh	Avoid	¾		Tbsp. (15g); 11g in total.
Pomegranate, fresh (arils-seed/juice sacs)	Avoid	2		Tbsp. (15g); 30g in total.
Quince, fresh	Free			Free of sorbitol.
Raisins, uncooked	Avoid	½		Portion (40g); 20g in total.
Rambutan, canned in syrup	Free			Free of sorbitol.
Raspberries, fresh, red	Avoid	1½		Portion (140g); 210g in total.
Rhubarb, fresh	Free			Free of sorbitol.
Rose hips	Free			Free of sorbitol.
Santa Claus melon	Free			Free of sorbitol.
Sapodilla, fresh	Free			Free of sorbitol.
Sour cherries, fresh	Avoid	½		Tbsp. (15g); 8g in total.

Fruit	SORBITOL Stand.		SORBITOL Low sensitivity amount
Soursop (guanabana), fresh	Free		Free of sorbitol.
Strawberries, fresh	Avoid	¼	Portion (140g); 35g in total.
Sweet cherries, fresh	Avoid	¼	Tbsp. (15g); 4g in total.
Watermelon, fresh	Nearly free		Nearly free of sorbitol

3.7.2 Vegetables

Vegetables	SORBITOL Stand.		SORBITOL Low sensitivity amount
Alfalfa sprouts	Free		Free of sorbitol.
Artichoke, globe raw	Avoid	23¾	Tbsp. (15g); 356g in total.
Arugula, raw	Free		Free of sorbitol.
Asparagus, raw	Avoid	9¾	Portion (85g); 829g in total.
Avocado, green skin, Florida type	Free		Free of sorbitol.
Bamboo shoots, canned and drained	Free		Free of sorbitol.
Beets, raw	Avoid	3¼	Portion (85g); 276g in total.
Black beans, cooked from dried	Free		Free of sorbitol.
Black olives	Avoid	33¼	Portion (15g); 499g in total.
Bok choy, raw	Avoid	23½	Portion (85g); 1998g in total.
Boston Market® sweet corn	Avoid	4	Portion (85g); 340g in total.
Broccoflower (green cauliflower), cooked from fresh	Free		Free of sorbitol.
Broccoli, raw	Free		Free of sorbitol.
Brown mushrooms (Italian or Crimini mushrooms), raw	Avoid	¾	Tbsp. (15g); 11g in total.
Brussels sprouts, cooked from fresh	Free		Free of sorbitol.
Butternut squash	Free		Free of sorbitol.

Vegetables	SORBITOL Stand.		SORBITOL Low sensitivity amount	
Cabbage, green, cooked	Avoid	58¾	Portion (85g); 4994g in total.
Cabbage, red, cooked	Free		Free of sorbitol.
Cabbage, savoy, raw	Avoid	39	Portion (85g); 3315g in total.
Carrots, cooked from fresh	Avoid	½	Portion (85g); 43g in total.
Carrots, raw	Avoid	¾	Piece (61g); 46g in total.
Cauliflower, cooked from frozen	Avoid	2½	Portion (85g); 213g in total.
Celeriac (celery root), cooked from fresh	Avoid	¾	Tbsp. (15g); 11g in total.
Celery, cooked	Avoid	1	Tbsp. (15g); 15g in total.
Chard, raw or blanched, marinated in oil	Free		Free of sorbitol.
Chayote squash, cooked	Free		Free of sorbitol.
Chestnuts, boiled, steamed	Avoid	6	Portion (30g); 180g in total.
Chicory coffee powder, unprepared	Avoid	8¾	Portion (2g); 18g in total.
Chicory greens, raw	Avoid	39	Portion (85g); 3315g in total.
Coleslaw, with apples and raisins, mayo dressing	Avoid	½	Portion (100g); 50g in total.
Coleslaw, with pineapple, mayo dressing	Avoid	3¾	Portion (100g); 375g in total.
Collards, raw	Free		Free of sorbitol.

Vegetables	SORBITOL Stand.		SORBITOL Low sensitivity amount	
Cucumber, raw, with peel	Avoid	1		Portion (85g); 85g in total.
Cucumber, raw, without peel	Avoid	1		Portion (85g); 85g in total.
Eggplant, cooked	Avoid	2½		Portion (85g); 213g in total.
Endive, curly, raw	Avoid	3		Portion (85g); 255g in total.
Enoki mushrooms, raw	Avoid	¾		Tbsp. (15g); 11g in total.
Fennel bulb, raw	Avoid	2		Portion (85g); 170g in total.
Garbanzo beans (chickpeas), canned, drained	Avoid	1		Portion (90g); 90g in total.
Garlic, fresh	Free			Free of sorbitol.
Ginger root, raw	Free			Free of sorbitol.
Green beans (string beans), cooked from fresh	Free			Free of sorbitol.
Green bell peppers	Free			Free of sorbitol.
Green olives	Avoid	18		Portion (15g); 270g in total.
Green tomato, raw	Avoid	¾		Portion (85g); 64g in total.
Grits (polenta), regular cooking	Free			Free of sorbitol.
Hot chili peppers, green, cooked from fresh	Free			Free of sorbitol.
Hot chili peppers, red, cooked from fresh	Free			Free of sorbitol.

Vegetables	SORBITOL Stand.		SORBITOL Low sensitivity amount	
Hubbard squash	Free			Free of sorbitol.
Jerusalem artichoke (sunchoke), raw	Free			Free of sorbitol.
Kale, raw	Avoid	¾		Portion (85g); 64g in total.
Kelp, raw	Free			Free of sorbitol.
Kidney beans, cooked from dried	Free			Free of sorbitol.
Kohlrabi, cooked	Avoid	13		Portion (85g); 1105g in total.
Leeks, leafs	Avoid	¼		Portion (85g); 21g in total.
Leeks, root	Avoid	2¼		Tbsp. (15g); 34g in total.
Leeks, whole	Avoid	¼		Portion (85g); 21g in total.
Lentils, cooked from dried	Free			Free of sorbitol.
Lettuce, Boston, bibb or butterhead	Avoid	19½		Portion (85g); 1658g in total.
Lettuce, green leaf	Avoid	16¾		Portion (85g); 1424g in total.
Lettuce, iceberg	Avoid	19½		Portion (85g); 1658g in total.
Lettuce, red leaf	Avoid	19½		Portion (85g); 1658g in total.
Lettuce, romaine or cos	Avoid	16¾		Portion (85g); 1424g in total.
Lima beans, cooked from dried	Free			Free of sorbitol.

Vegetables	SORBITOL Stand.		SORBITOL Low sensitivity amount	
Lotus root, cooked	Free			Free of sorbitol.
Maitake mushrooms, raw	Avoid	¾		Tbsp. (15g); 11g in total.
Morel mushrooms, raw	Avoid	¾		Tbsp. (15g); 11g in total.
Mung bean sprouts, cooked from fresh	Avoid	16¾		Portion (85g); 1424g in total.
Mung beans, cooked from dried	Free			Free of sorbitol.
Mushrooms, batter dipped or breaded	Avoid	¼		Portion (70g); 18g in total.
Okra, raw	Free			Free of sorbitol.
Onion, white, yellow or red, raw	Avoid	6		Tbsp. (15g); 90g in total.
Oyster mushrooms, raw	Avoid	¼		Portion (85g); 21g in total.
Parsnip, cooked	Free			Free of sorbitol.
Pickled beets	Avoid	15		Portion (30g); 450g in total.
Portabella mushrooms, cooked from fresh	Avoid	½		Tbsp. (15g); 8g in total.
Purslane, raw	Free			Free of sorbitol.
Radicchio, raw	Free			Free of sorbitol.
Radish, raw	Avoid	1		Portion (85g); 85g in total.
Rutabaga, raw or blanched, marinated in oil mixture	Free			Free of sorbitol.

Vegetables	SORBITOL Stand.		SORBITOL Low sensitivity amount	
Sauerkraut	Avoid	¾	Tbsp. (15g); 11g in total.
Scallop squash	Free		Free of sorbitol.
Shallot, raw	Free		Free of sorbitol.
Shiitake mushrooms, cooked	Avoid	½	Tbsp. (15g); 8g in total.
Snow peas (edible pea pods), cooked from fresh	Free		Free of sorbitol.
Sour pickles	Avoid	4¼	Portion (30g); 128g in total.
Soybean sprouts, raw	Avoid	½	Portion (85g); 43g in total.
Soybeans, cooked from dried	Avoid	3	Tbsp. (15g); 45g in total.
Spaghetti squash	Free		Free of sorbitol.
Spinach, cooked from fresh	Avoid	13	Portion (85g); 1105g in total.
Split pea sprouts, cooked	Free		Free of sorbitol.
Straw mushrooms, canned, drained	Avoid	¼	Portion (85g); 21g in total.
Summer squash, cooked from fresh	Free		Free of sorbitol.
Sun-dried tomatoes, oil pack, drained	Avoid	¾	Tbsp. (15g); 11g in total.
Sweet potato, boiled	Free		Free of sorbitol.
Tempeh	Avoid	½	Portion (85g); 43g in total.

Vegetables	SORBITOL Stand.		SORBITOL Low sensitivity amount	
Tomato, cooked from fresh	☹	Avoid	¾	Portion (85g); 64g in total.
Turnip, cooked	☹	Avoid	2½	Portion (85g); 213g in total.
Wax beans (yellow beans), canned, drained	☺	Free	☺	Free of sorbitol.
Winter melon (waxgourd or chinese preserving melon)	☺	Free	☺	Free of sorbitol.
Winter type (dark green or orange) squash, cooked	☺	Free	☺	Free of sorbitol.
Yams, sweet potato type, boiled	☺	Free	☺	Free of sorbitol.
Yellow bell pepper, raw	☺	Free	☺	Free of sorbitol.
Yellow tomato, raw	☹	Avoid	1	Portion (85g); 85g in total.

3.8 Ice cream

Ice cream	SORBITOL Stand.	SORBITOL Low sensitivity amount
Ben & Jerry's® Ice Cream, Brownie Batter	Nearly free	Nearly free of sorbitol
Ben & Jerry's® Ice Cream, Chocolate Chip Cookie Dough	Free	Free of sorbitol.
Ben & Jerry's® Ice Cream, Chubby Hubby®	Free	Free of sorbitol.
Ben & Jerry's® Ice Cream, Chunky Monkey®	Nearly free	Nearly free of sorbitol
Ben & Jerry's® Ice Cream, Half Baked	Free	Free of sorbitol.
Ben & Jerry's® Ice Cream, Karamel Sutra®	Free	Free of sorbitol.
Ben & Jerry's® Ice Cream, New York Super Fudge Chunk®	Nearly free	Nearly free of sorbitol
Ben & Jerry's® Ice Cream, One Sweet Whirled	Free	Free of sorbitol.
Ben & Jerry's® Ice Cream, Peanut Butter Cup	Free	Free of sorbitol.
Ben & Jerry's® Ice Cream, Phish Food®	Free	Free of sorbitol.
Ben & Jerry's® Ice Cream, Vanilla For A Change	Free	Free of sorbitol.
Breyers® Ice Cream, Natural Vanilla, Lactose Free	Free	Free of sorbitol.
Dreyer's® Grand Ice Cream, Chocolate	Nearly free	Nearly free of sorbitol
Dreyer's® No Sugar Added Ice Cream, Triple Chocolate	Avoid	Avoid consumption!

Ice cream	SORBITOL Stand.		SORBITOL Low sensitivity amount
Drumstick® (sundae cone)	Nearly free		Nearly free of sorbitol
Frozen fruit juice Bar	Avoid	4½	Piece (77g); 347g in total.
Haagen-Dazs® Desserts Extraordinaire Ice Cream, Creme Brulee	Free		Free of sorbitol.
Haagen-Dazs® Frozen Yogurt, chocolate or coffee flavors	Nearly free		Nearly free of sorbitol
Haagen-Dazs® Frozen Yogurt, vanilla or other flavors	Free		Free of sorbitol.
Haagen-Dazs® Ice Cream, Bailey's Irish Cream	Nearly free		Nearly free of sorbitol
Haagen-Dazs® Ice Cream, Black Walnut	Free		Free of sorbitol.
Haagen-Dazs® Ice Cream, Butter Pecan	Free		Free of sorbitol.
Haagen-Dazs® Ice Cream, Cherry Vanilla	Free		Free of sorbitol.
Haagen-Dazs® Ice Cream, Chocolate	Nearly free		Nearly free of sorbitol
Haagen-Dazs® Ice Cream, Coffee	Nearly free		Nearly free of sorbitol
Haagen-Dazs® Ice Cream, Cookies & Cream	Free		Free of sorbitol.
Haagen-Dazs® Ice Cream, Mango	Free		Free of sorbitol.
Haagen-Dazs® Ice Cream, Pistachio	Free		Free of sorbitol.
Haagen-Dazs® Ice Cream, Rocky Road	Nearly free		Nearly free of sorbitol

Ice cream	SORBITOL Stand.		SORBITOL Low sensitivity amount
Haagen-Dazs® Ice Cream, Rocky Road	☺	Nearly free	☺ Nearly free of sorbitol
Haagen-Dazs® Ice Cream, Strawberry	☺	Free	☺ Free of sorbitol.
Haagen-Dazs® Ice Cream, Vanilla Chocolate Chip	☺	Free	☺ Free of sorbitol.
Ice cream sandwich	☺	Free	☺ Free of sorbitol.
Ice cream, light, no sugar added, with aspartame, vanilla or other flavors (include chocolate chip)	☹	Avoid	¼ Tsp. (5g); 1g in total.
Popsicle	☺	Free	☺ Free of sorbitol.
Popsicle, sugar free	☺	Free	☺ Free of sorbitol.
Sorbet, chocolate	☺	Free	☺ Free of sorbitol.
Sorbet, coconut	☺	Free	☺ Free of sorbitol.
Sorbet, fruit	☺	Free	☺ Free of sorbitol.

3.9 Ingredients

Ingredients	SORBITOL Stand.	SORBITOL Low sensitivity amount
Baking powder	☺ Free	☺ Free of sorbitol.
Barley flour	☺ Free	☺ Free of sorbitol.
Lemon peel	☺ Free	☺ Free of sorbitol.
Orange peel	☺ Free	☺ Free of sorbitol.
Rye flour, in recipes not containing yeast	☺ Free	☺ Free of sorbitol.
Semolina flour	☺ Free	☺ Free of sorbitol.
Spelt flour	☺ Free	☺ Free of sorbitol.
Streusel topping, crumb	☺ Free	☺ Free of sorbitol.
Wheat bran, unprocessed	☺ Free	☺ Free of sorbitol.
White all-purpose flour, un-enriched	☺ Free	☺ Free of sorbitol.
White whole wheat flour	☺ Free	☺ Free of sorbitol.

Glossary

Abbreviation	Meaning
EFSA	European Food Safety Authority.
FDA	Food and Drug Administration.
Fructans	Quickly fermentable carbohydrates that are contained in grain products for example. Included in this group are inulin, kestose and nystose.
Fructose	Oligosaccharide that is primarily contained in fruit.
Galactans	Quickly fermentable carbohydrates that are contained in beans, cabbage, lentils and peas for example (raffinose and stachyose).
Hereditary fructose intolerance	This disease is rare. If you are affected, fructose has a poisonous effect on you. Only a specialist can find out if you are affected and you have to check it before doing a test for fructose intolerance, as it could otherwise be lethal.
Irritable bowel	Definition of this book: an irritable bowel is one that reacts much more intensely to indigestions than it is commonly the case. The presence of trigger cubes in the intestine triggers the symptoms.
Lactose	Oligosaccharide that is primarily contained in dairy products.
Meal	One of three main meals of a given day. The first meal happens at about 7 am the second one at about 1 pm and the third one at about 7 pm. Hence, between each meal there has to be a gap of about six hours in order to avoid overloading your enzyme workers. The tolerable portion sizes refer to this definition of a meal.
NCC	Nutrition Coordination Center of the University of Minnesota.

Abbreviation	Meaning
Sensitivity level	Aside from the standard level, you can use multipliers to determine portion sizes in case you are less sensitive. In the LAXIBA app, we have calculated the tolerable amounts for you. Before increasing your portion sizes to fit another level, you should do a level test to check, if you can tolerate the higher load. There are four levels, see Chapter 3.1.1.
Sorbitol	Sugar alcohol that bacteria ferment in the large intestine and thereby causes you symptoms. In this book, sorbitol refers to all nine sugar-alcohols that may cause your symptoms. See as well: sugar-alcohols.
Standard	Portion sizes in this column are based on the usual sensitivity in case of an intolerance towards sorbitol, i.e. as long as you consume less than the stated maximum amount for level 0, you are likely to be untroubled by symptoms from it. Note that if you consume the maximum portion size for a food at a meal, you cannot eat any other foods that contain sorbitol at that meal. To combine two foods that contain a certain cube you have to reduce the stated portion sizes accordingly, e.g. by dividing both by two.
Sugar-alcohols	These are contained in some fruit, like apples. Moreover, they are part of many diabetic, dietary and light products as well as chewing gums and mints. They are not contained in stevia. Part of the group of sugar-alcohols besides sorbitol are erythritol, inositol, isomalt, lactitol, maltitol, mannitol, pinitol and xylitol.
Trigger(cube)s	Carbohydrates that fermented in the intestine. To this group belong oligosaccharides (fructose, fructans and galactans, lactose) and sugar-alcohols (like sorbitol).

4

ADVANCED PROCEDURES

4.1 Level test

	Level test tasks	✔
1	You filled out the symptom test sheet for the status quo check.	✔
2	You asked your doctor to refer you to a specialist to do a breath test (if available).	✔
3	You performed the three-week introductory diet and found an improvement to your symptoms at the efficiency check (otherwise get *THE IBS NAVIGATOR* and find your trigger). If no breath test was available, you performed the substitute test.	✔
4	Now you convince a partner to help you with your tests. Alternatively, you book a personal trainer at *https://laxiba.com/trainer*. The partner will mix your test liquids and interpret your symptom test sheets. You can count on their confidentiality, credibility and availability.	
5	You finished all of the tests, during which your testing partner adhered to the instructions on page 171, and you acted according to the flowchart on page 182.	
6	Finish: You talked your result over with your testing partner, and adapted your serving sizes to your sensitivity level.	

Each human differs in the amount he or she can stomach of each trigger. Even in healthy humans the tolerated amount of sorbitol, for example, fluctuates between 5g and about 25 g. Moreover, the amount consumed at once for the breath or substitute test is higher than what you would consume in a typical meal. Hence, if your enzyme-workers were able to cope with that amount—you were spared from symptoms after consuming the test does—you can be proud of them, and you can give them a positive interim report: They have mastered all tasks for sorbitol with flying colors.

If your crew has ached at the dose, at that point all we know is that the extreme test amount has been too much for them. What it does not mean is that the standard portion sizes used in this book are the highest load your enzyme workers can take. Where is your personal threshold up to which you will not have symptoms? To determine it, you use the level test described in the following. With it, you challenge your enzyme worker gradually and check your sensitivity. With each step, you increase the consumption amount of sorbitol up to the point at which your enzyme workers ask for a pay raise. The flowchart on page 182 depicts the procedure.

For the level test, you ideally have a test partner preparing the test liquids for you and checking the results. If you have one, only let your partner read the instructions on the pages 168 onward. To increase the reliability, you test each level twice. Otherwise, chance could cause something else to trigger your symptom. Should you consider the matter too private and rather not have someone else included, follow the instructions for self-testers you find on those pages.

Start your test week three days before the test day, as symptoms may occur as many as three days after you consume sorbitol containing foods, and you want to start the check uninfluenced from "old" symptoms. On the days before the test, eat according to your current level. Your current level is the one that you tolerated during the previous test and retest. Initially, it is the level 0 amount in the serving size tables of Chapter 3.

How to run a test week

Day 1–3 before the test day	On the test day	Day 1–3 after
Your cube consumption should undercut your current sorbitol levels by as narrow a margin as possible, but do not force yourself to eat more of anything than you want. If you do not feel as well on the morning of the test day as you did at the end of the introductory diet, reschedule the test until you do.	Fill out the symptom test sheet on the test day and its three subsequent days.	
	At breakfast, lunch and dinner consume the level dose and apart from that avoid sorbitol-containing foods.	Eat accoding to the level on day 1-3 before the test. Hence, if you test level 1 go back down to level 0.

Acceleration option: Perform the tests right after one another. Three days after the last test day, begin the next test day and thus save the three days described in the column on the left.

You do not have to fill out the symptom test sheet during the days leading up to the test (page 25). Instead, you can use the efficiency check sheet as your reference, but from the day of the test to the third day after it, document your symptoms (unless you determine an intolerance earlier).

When your testing partner confirms you have an intolerance, the level test is over. You can find the precise procedure in the flowcharts in Section 4.2. For procedural reasons, wait until after you have repeated the test before trying to interpret the results.

How to handle symptoms

After noting discomforts that were so severe that you told your test collaborate you malabsorbed the load, drink water (up to three liters per day are usually healthy) and take a walk to reduce your symptoms.

Information for your level test partner:

My calculated K.O. threshold grade is:

If you want to use the mathematical Option B, presented at the end of this Chapter or are using our downloadable tool, enter your K.O.-grade from the efficiency check above or give your partner the filled out excel sheets. Important: disregard triggers that you can stomach—you can consume products containing them just as you did before. Background: if your estimated symptom grade (lid value) after a level test is lower or equal to the estimate K.O. grade, you have tolerated the test load and thereby the level and otherwise you have not.

 ## Summary

As part of the strategy, you first performed the introductory diet to find out, if the diet did reduce your symptoms after all. If it had an effect, you can go on to determine your individual sensitivity to avoid unnecessary restrictions.

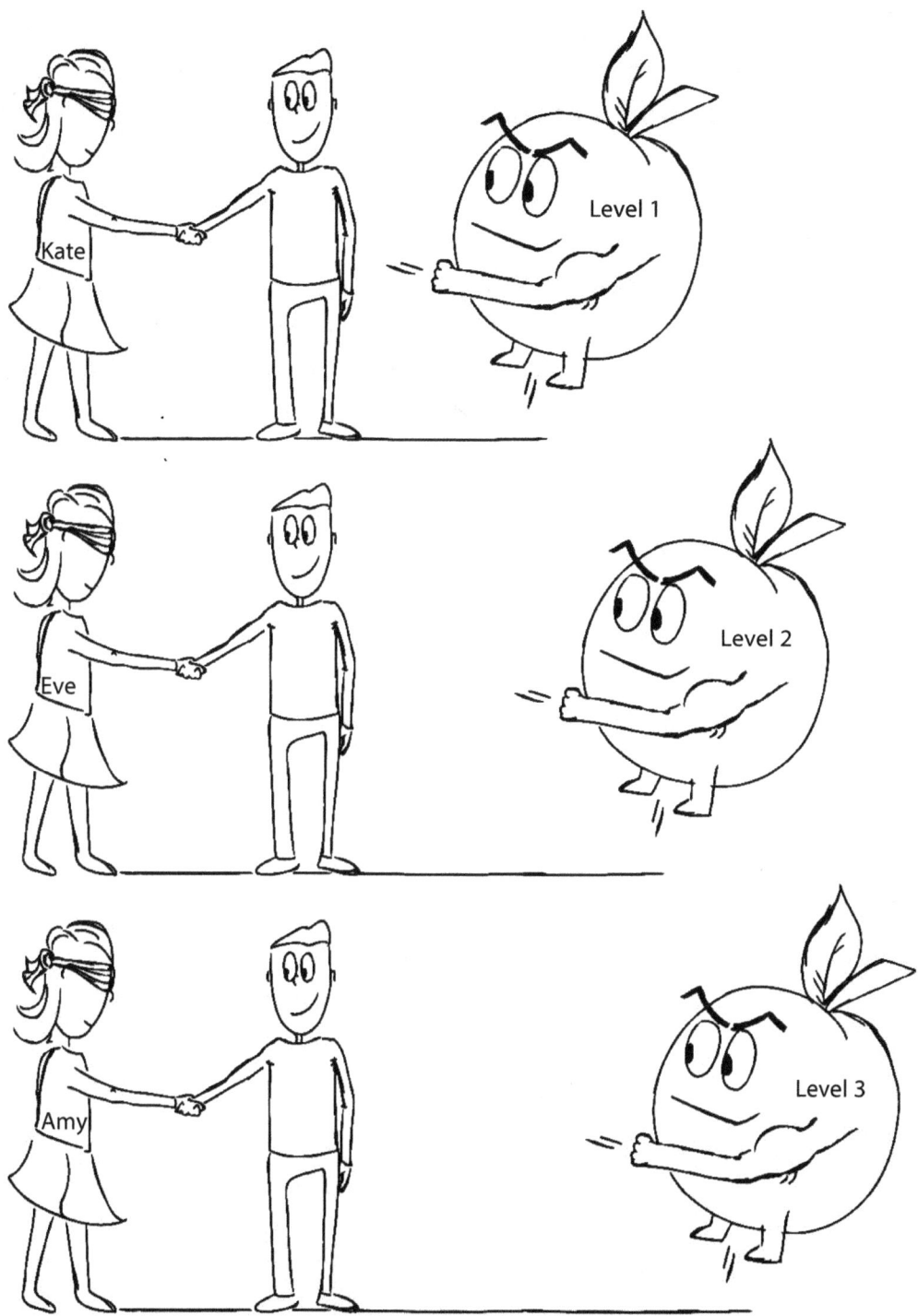

Everyone's sensitivity level is different.

STOP: The following pages are for only your testing partner to read, as they contain information regarding procedural safety—unless you want to do the test alone! Your partner's instructions will depend on your reactions; if you know how your partner is assessing you, you may alter your behavior and distort the results. Continue reading on page 182 to learn about the procedure underlying your partner's tolerance statements. Before and after the three pages for your testing partner are four empty pages. Thus, you can flick back from the end of the book to arrive at page 182 without reading them.

The **instructions** for your testing **partner** follow on page **171**. As the **reader** of the book, you should leave them **unread**, to **produce** a **more accurate** test **result**. Hence, open a new page that is farther **ahead** and then **flick back** to page **182**.

The **instructions** for your testing **partner** follow on page **171**. As the **reader** of the book, you should leave them **unread**, to **produce** a **more accurate** test **result**. Hence, open a new page that is much farther **ahead** and then **flick back** to page **182**.

The **instructions** for your testing **partner** follow on page **171**. As the **reader** of the book, you should leave them **unread**, to **produce** a **more accurate** test **result**. Hence, open a new page that is much farther **ahead** and then **flick back** to page **182**.

The **instructions** for your testing **partner** follow on page **171**. As the **reader** of the book, you should leave them **unread**, to **produce** a **more accurate** test **result**. Hence, open a new page that is much farther **ahead** and then **flick back** to page **182**.

Your friend needs your help! Instructions for testing partners:

You are not the testing partner but the aggrieved party? In case, I caught you! However, of course you also find instructions how to conduct the test yourself. If have a testing partner these lines are not for you, would you please finally move on to page 182!

Now we are in private. Your friend cannot stomach sorbitol, a common food ingredient, and wants to find out about the personal tolerance limit. Unfortunately, a placebo effect is quite common in this test. Your role in this test is critical for avoiding a false result. You are going to do two rounds per level, each test taking about a week. On one of the two days, you are going to hand out a placebo mix instead of the real one. Your friend does not know about the placebo. Just say that the double test is required to get valid results, as you also have to keep track of certain behaviors she or he might exhibit. IMPORTANT: Keep quiet about the placebo until **all** tests are done (use the flowchart on page 182) and you have talked the results over. Waiting until the end of that final discussion is important, as your friend may want to test another level as well. Between two test days are three monitoring days and three regeneration days. Here is what you need: a beaker, a letter scale, and three 0.5 L bottles. Also, instruct your friend to stop taking another bottle if the symptoms after drinking one are already indicating that the load was too much.

> **Note in case you have to do the test without a testing partner**: Prepare the required test bottles on the eve before the test. Make the real and the placebo mix in an equal looking 1-liter-bottle with a non-transparent plastic label (the foil around the bottle on which the brand name shows up). If you use milk, make sure it is still usable for at least two weeks. Now use a pen and write placebo on a colored memo, fold it twice to form a smaller square and put it behind the label of the bottle with the placebo mix. On another note in the same color, you write real mix and put it behind the label of the other bottle. Then you put sticky tape around the tags. Then put both bottles into a non-transparent box that is longer, wider and higher than the bottles. Close it and then turn it around ten times. Thus, you have successfully outwitted yourself: put the bottles in the fridge! On the next morning, you take out one of the bottles, mark it with 1 and drink one third of the mixture in the morning, one third at lunchtime and the rest of the evening (you use one bottle with the daily amount instead of three here, according to the first column of the following tables).

If you find yourself trying to spy at the memo, give yourself a slap on the finger. After the three days following it, where you observed your symptoms, you repeat the test with the other bottle. Again, no fiddling with the label! You have to wait with that until the three observance days of the second bottle are over, too. Now check, how you stomached the placebo versus the real mix.

If your friend has not given you the substances for the test solution, you can order them online or from a pharmacy. You can also ask your pharmacist to weigh the amounts you need. From test to test, increase the level amounts according to the table on the following page. Begin with the level 1 amount. Before repeating the test, note whether you first handed out the real or placebo mix and the result. Ideally, you should ask for the symptom test sheet and write down L for reaL and A for plAcebo as well as the result. Then, keep all of the info sheets for the final discussion of all tests. If your friend has given you the K-grade, you can calculate the tolerance (see row L on page 184). If the L-grade is greater than or equal to K, this indicates an intolerance. There are three possible cases after each double test:

Case 1: Neither the placebo nor the real mix causes the symptoms to worsen, i.e., your friend can stomach the amounts of the ingredient, and you can test the next level. Tell her/him that.

Case 2: Only the real mix causes the symptoms to worsen, i.e., your friend is intolerant for the amount. The test series is over, and you can tell your friend.

Case 3: The placebo mix causes symptoms to worsen. Regardless of whether or not the real mix causes symptoms to worsen, as well, repeat the test with the same amount, starting with the placebo mix, but tell her that you reduced the amount to half of the dose. If your friend still reports an intolerance, abort the test and tell her/him that s/he has an intolerance for the amount, and the old levels remain current.

After the test and retest of the first level of the ingredient, continue according to the level test flowchart on pp. 182. On the eve of one of the two test days, hand out three bottles with the real mix, and on the other one, three bottles with the placebo. At breakfast, lunch and dinner your friend drinks one bottle. You can find the mixtures for each level in the following explanation and table.

In the **left column** find the respective **level** and the **total amount** of substances per day, as it is easier to mix the **daily amount in one load** and **then divide** it among the **three bottles**. In the two columns on the right, find the amounts per bottle for the real/placebo substance. Required: 10g of sorbitol and table sugar. Mix the amounts with 200 mL of water and add a little bit of vanilla extract (**v.**). Important: you should not dilute the contents:

Level, real/placebo mix **per day**+600 mL water	Real (R) 3 × 200 mL water bottle with	Placebo (P) 3 × 200 mL water bottle with
Level 1, 0.3 R/0.2 P, 1 tsp. **v.**	0.1g sorbitol 3 drops of **v.**	0.06g sugar 3 drops of **v.**
Level 2, 1.2 R/0.7 P, 1 tsp. **v.**	0.4g sorbitol 3 drops of **v.**	0.24g sugar 3 drops of **v.**
Level 3, 3 R/1.26 P, 1 tsp. **v.**	0.7g sorbitol 3 drops of **v.**	0.42g sugar 3 drops of **v.**

Thank you very much for your support! Even if you have to overcome scruples to knowingly trick your friend… You do not? Well then, enjoy the white lie for good reason!

The **instructions** for your testing **partner** begin on page **171**. As the **reader** of the book, you should leave them **unread**, to **produce** a **more accurate** test **result**. The book resumes on page 182.

The **instructions** for your testing **partner** begin on page **171**. As the **reader** of the book, you should leave them **unread**, to **produce** a **more accurate** test **result**. The book resumes on page 182.

The **instructions** for your testing **partner** begin on page **171**. As the **reader** of the book, you should leave them **unread**, to **produce** a **more accurate** test **result**. The book resumes on page 182.

The **instructions** for your testing **partner** begin on page **171**. As the **reader** of the book, you should leave them **unread**, to **produce** a **more accurate** test **result**.

4.2 Symptom-based test process

The following flow chart shows you the next step, depending on your reaction to the test load. Remember, if you have symptoms after taking the first of three test loads on a test day, abort the test—as this shows that the tested sensitivity level is too high, and there is no point in tantalizing yourself.

You start the test with the first field of the flow chart. The next step always depends on your test result. If you did not stomach a load, the test is over, and you should stick to the level below, which you did tolerate—at the beginning this is the standard amount in the tables in Chapter 3.

All statements assume that you want to perform the level test to the highest level. However, maybe, it is enough to you to know if you tolerate the next level, in the case just stop after the first test. If you do tolerate more than the standard level, note your level next to the multipliers, see Chapter 3.1.1. You will also be able to select your level when using our mobile phone application. Attention: During the combined level tests, you must not pass any level amount that holds for one of your triggers that you do not check at the time as this may otherwise distort the result. If it does happen, you have to repeat the check.

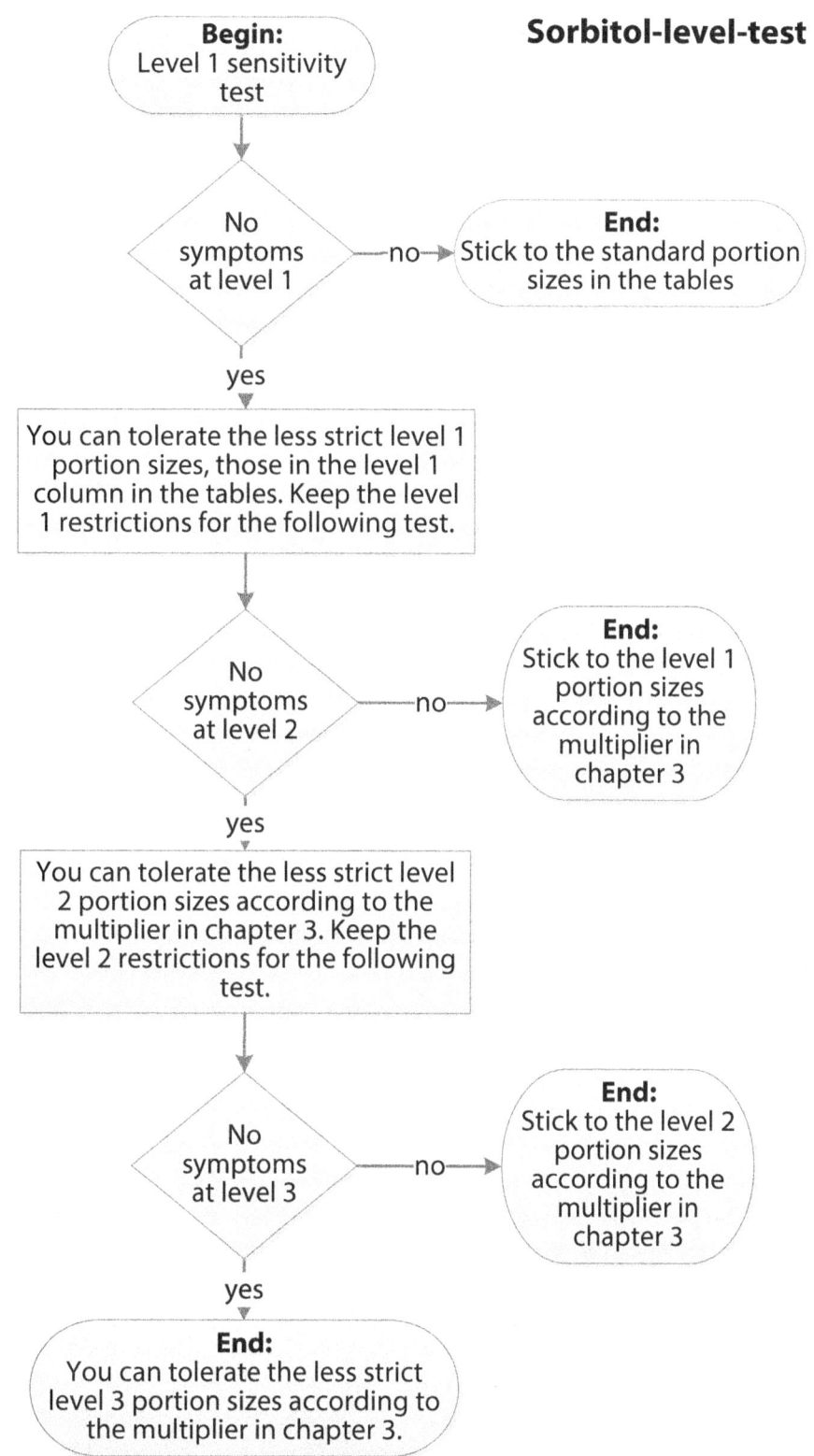

4.3 Test result calculation table

You have two calculation options: option **A** is slightly simpler than option **B**. Real cracks immediately start with **B**. **B** saves time at any further check, and you get a statement on your tolerance. [4]

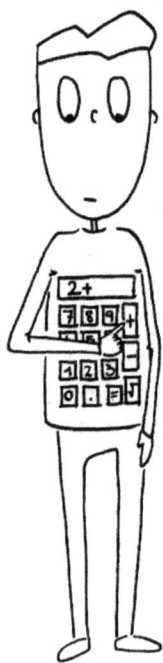

---

[4] From a statistical point of view the survey is slim and the result vague.

4.3.1 The efficiency check calculation table

You use the following table and enter the total intensity of bloating of the respective day into the row **A**. Into the first four cells of that row, you enter the results of the **efficiency check days**, i.e. the last days of your introductory diet. Into the remaining four fields of that row, you enter the values of the **status-quo-days** (the four days before starting your introductory diet, hence, before reducing your trigger consumption).

Calculation option A: Determine $A1$ = total stool grade at the first day of your efficiency check, i.e. your grade in the morning (you calculate your stool grade by multiplying your stool value by the number of defecations you had in the morning) plus the grade at lunchtime plus the grade at the evening. Likewise, you proceed with all other **A**-numbers. Afterward, you determine the **B**-numbers: $B1 = A1$ plus the bloating grade at the first efficiency-check-day plus the pain grade on that day. You calculate $B2$ likewise with the grades for day 2 and so on. Next, you calculate $C2$ and afterward $D2$, which is the average of the status-quo-check-days. To interpret the result, you compare $D2$ with the highest day-grade of the efficiency-check-days, the highest grade of the group $B1$ to $B4$. When checking the success of the introductory diet, it holds that the greater $D2$ lies above the maximum grade of the group the more likely it is that the introductory diet was successful in lowering your symptoms.

Calculation Option B: You calculate $A1$ to $A8$ as well as $B1$ to $B8$ according to the calculation option **A**. Afterward, you estimate $C1$ and $D1$, as well as $C2$ and $D2$ and proceed with the steps described in the table up to K. To interpret the result you compare the $D2$-value with the K-value, i.e. the K. O.[5] threshold grade. At the introductory diet, it holds that: If $D2$ is bigger or equal to the K-grade; this indicates that the diet successfully lowered your symptoms.

If the diet fails, however, get *THE IBS NAVIGATOR* and take the substitute test for fructans and galactans or check alternative triggers as described there.

---

[5] K = if L tops this K.-O.-threshold, the level test amount is too much for your enzyme workers.

	Efficiency check day-				Status-quo-check-day before introductory diet			
	1:	2:	3:	4:	1:	2:	3:	4:
A	A1	A3	A3	A4	A5	A6	A7	A8
	Enter the total stool grade for each day into the A-cells							
B	B1	B2	B3	B4	B5	B6	B7	B8
	B5 = stool- + bloating- + pain grade on status-quo-check-day 1							
C	C1	C1 = B1 + B2 + B3 + B4 Sum of cells B1 to B4							C2
		C2 = B5 + B6 + B7 + B8 Sum of cells B5 to B8							
D	D1	D1 = C1 ÷ 4 Divide your result in cell C1 by 4							D2
		D2 = C2 ÷ 4 Divide your result in cell C2 by 4							
E	E1	E2	E3	E4	E1 = B1 - D1, E2 = B2 - D1 etc. To calculate E1, subtract D1 from B1. Negative results are possible.			
F	F1	F2	F3	F4	F1 = E1 x E1, F2 = E2 x E2 etc. To calculate F1, multiply E1 by itself. As minus times minus is plus, all results are positive.			
G	G	G = F1 + F2 + F3 + F4 Add your results of the cells F1 to F4						
H	H	H = G ÷ 4 Divide G by 4						
I	I	I = Take the root of H Take the root of your result in H. On your calculator the root symbol looks like this: √.						
J	J	J = I x 2 Multiply I by 2						
K	K	K = J + D1 Add the result of cell J to the one in cell D1. The K-grade is the K. O. threshold grade as the success of the introductory diet depends on it. The diet lowered your symptoms if D2 is bigger than K (D2 > K). In addition, you can assess the success of the sensitivity level test with it. You tolerated the tested level if L is not bigger than K (L ≤ K). Please transfer the K-grade to the level test table.						

1. Efficiency check calculation with page 27-28 values

	Efficiency-check-day-				Status-quo-check-day before introductory diet			
	1:	2:	3:	4:	1:	2:	3:	4:
A	A1 3	A3 2	A3 3	A4 2	A5 16	A6 14	A7 12	A8 14
	Enter the total stool grade for each day into the A-cells							
B	B1 9	B2 8	B3 11	B4 8	B5 30	B6 30	B7 31	B8 28
	B5 = stool- + bloating- + pain grade on status-quo-check-day 1							
C	C1 36	C1 = B1 + B2 + B3 + B4 Sum of cells B1 to B4 C2 = B5 + B6 + B7 + B8 Sum of cells B5 to B8					C2 119	
D	D1 9	D1 = C1 ÷ 4 Divide your result in cell C1 by 4 D2 = C2 ÷ 4 Divide your result in cell C2 by 4					D2 29.75	
E	E1 0	E2 -1	E3 2	E4 -1	E1 = B1 - D1, E2 = B2 - D1 etc. To calculate E1, subtract D1 from B1. Negative results are possible.			
F	F1 0	F2 1	F3 4	F4 1	F1 = E1 x E1, F2 = E2 x E2 etc. To calculate F1, multiply E1 by itself. As minus times minus is plus, all results are positive.			
G	G 6	G = F1 + F2 + F3 + F4 Add your results of the cells F1 to F4						
H	H 1.5	H = G ÷ 4 Divide G by 4						
I	I 1.22	I = Take the root of H Take the root of your result in H. On your calculator the root symbol looks like this: $\sqrt{}$.						
J	J 2.45	J = I x 2 Multiply I by 2						
K	K 11.45	K = J + D1 Add the result of cell J to the one in cell D1. The K-grade is called K. O. threshold grade as the success of the introductory diet (D2 > K) and the sensitivity level test (L ≤ K) depend on it.						

Calculation method A

D2 is 29.75 and thus way larger than the highest day grade, 11, (B3) of the group B1 to B4, which indicates the success of the introductory diet.

Calculation method B

D2 = 29.75 is bigger than K = 11.45, and that shows the success of the diet. Had D2 been smaller or equal to K, get *THE IBS NAVIGATOR* and check other triggers.

4.3.2 The level test calculation table

Use the following table and enter the grades of the level test days. You only need to estimate the grades from the level test sheet (enter them into B5 to B8. If you used math option B, just enter the K value, and you are ready to determine your result. If you use math option A, you have to calculate D1. Having done the introductory diet is, of course, necessary.

Calculation option A: $A1$ = stool grade at the first efficiency-check-day, i.e. grade in the morning (multiply the stool value in the morning by the number of defecations you had in the morning) plus stool grade at lunchtime plus stool grade at the evening. Enter your total stool grade into the cell with the $A1$ in italic. Likewise, you proceed with all other **A**-Numbers. Afterward, estimate the **B-grades**: $B1 = A1$ plus total bloating grade plus total pain grade on the test day. You calculate $B2$ with the grades for the first day after the test day and so on. Next, you determine $C1$ and afterward $D1$, i.e. the average of the efficiency-check days. To interpret the result, compare $D1$ with the highest day grade of the level test days, $B5$ to $B8$. When checking the success of the diet, it holds that the much greater the largest day grade is compared to $D1$, the rather you did not tolerate the load of the tested sensitivity level. If that is the case, stick to the portion sizes of a lower sensitivity level.

Calculation option B: If you calculated K at the efficiency check—you should have as doing a level test before checking the efficiency of the diet makes no sense—just copy it to this table. Aside from it, all you need is to estimate $B1$ to $B8$ according to calculation option **A** and determine L. For the assessment, you compare the L-, i.e. the level grade with the K-grade, the K.-O.-threshold grade. It holds: if L is bigger than K, this means that the amount consumed during the test has triggered symptoms. Therefore, you should stick to the portion sizes of the sensitivity level below at which your symptoms improved. If L is lower than K, you tolerated the level amount and can have the less restricted diet according to that level. What is more, you can check an even higher sensitivity level if you want.

	Efficiency-check-day-				Level-test	day after test day-		
	1:	**2:**	**3:**	**4:**	**Test day**	**1:**	**2:**	**3:**
A	*A1*	*A3*	*A3*	*A4*	*A5*	*A6*	*A7*	*A8*
	Enter the total stool grade for each day into the A-cells							
B	*B1*	*B2*	*B3*	*B4*	*B5*	*B6*	*B7*	*B8*
	B5 = stool- + bloating- + pain grade on status-quo-check-day 1							
C	*C1*	*C1 = B1 + B2 + B3 + B4* Sum of the cells *B1* to *B4*						
D	*D1*	*D1 = C1 ÷ 4* Divide your results in cell *C1* by 4						
K	*K*	Please copy the K grade you estimated at the end of the introductory diet to this field. If you have not yet calculated it, do it now as described in the *efficiency-check-calculation-table*.						
L	*L*	*L* = is the biggest grade of the group: *B5, B6, B7, B8*. This group contains the results of the level test day (*B5*) and the three days following it (*B6* to *B8*). With the *L*-grade, you evaluate the current Level test. Assessment: *L > K*, if L is bigger than K, it means that the tested load for that level caused you symptoms and that you, therefore, should adjust your diet to a lower sensitivity level. *L ≤ K*, if L is lower or equal to K, it means that you tolerated the load of that level per meal.						

1. Level test calculation with the page 27-28 values

	Efficiency-check-day-				Level-test	day after test day-		
	1:	2:	3:	4:	Test day	1:	2:	3:
A	A1 3	A3 2	A3 3	A4 2	A5 16	A6 14	A7 12	A8 14
	Enter the total stool grade for each day into the A-cells							
B	B1 9	B2 8	B3 11	B4 8	B5 30	B6 30	B7 31	B8 28
	B5 = stool- + bloating- + pain grade on status-quo-check-day 1							
C	C1 36	C1 = B1 + B2 + B3 + B4 Sum of the cells B1 to B4						
D	D1 9	D1 = C1 ÷ 4 Divide your results in cell C1 by 4						
K	K 11.45	Please copy the K grade you estimated at the end of the introductory diet to this field. If you have not yet calculated it, do it now as described in the efficiency-check-calculation-table.						
L	L 31	L = is the biggest grade of the group: B5, B6, B7, B8. This group contains the results of the level test day (B5) and the three days following it (B6 to B8). With the L-grade, you evaluate the current Level test. Assessment: L > K, if L is bigger than K, it means that the tested load for that level caused you symptoms and that you, therefore, should adjust your diet to a lower sensitivity level. L ≤ K, if L is lower or equal to K, it means that you tolerated the load of that level per meal.						

Calculation method A

The highest total grade of a day of the group B5 to B8, B7 = 31 is way above D1 = 9, which indicates that you did not tolerate the level amount. If the highest grade of the group B5 to B8 had been smaller or equal to 9, you would have tolerated the sensitivity level amount and could have taken a less restricted diet according to the amounts of that level. Moreover, you could have tested the next level for people that are even less sensitive.

Calculation method B

As L = 31 is bigger than K = 11.45, you have not tolerated the level load of that trigger. Had L been smaller or equal to 11.45, you would have endured the level amount and could have followed the less strict diet for that level. Moreover, you could have tested the next higher tolerance level.

Sources

Ali, M., Rellos, P., & Cox, T. M. (1998). Heriditary fruktose intolerance. *Journal of Medical Genetics*, 35(5), 353-365.

American Cancer Society (2015). *Colorectal cancer and early detection*. Retrieved from: www.cancer.org/acs/groups/cis/documents/webcontent/003170-pdf.pdf.

Ananthakrishnan, A. N., Higuchi, L. M., Huang, E. S., Khalili, H., Richter, J. M., Fuchs, C. S., & Chan, A. T. (2012). Aspirin, nonsteroidal anti-inflammatory drug use, and risk for Crohn disease and ulcerative colitis: a cohort study. *Annals of Internal Medicine*, 156(5), 350-359.

Barrett, J. S., Gearry, R. B., Muir, J. G., Irving, P. M., Rose, R., Rosella, O., ... & Gibson, P. R. (2010). Dietary poorly absorbed, short-chain carbohydrates increase delivery of water and fermentable substrates to the proximal colon. *Alimentary Pharmacology & Therapeutics*, 31(8), 874-882.

Balasubramanya, N. N., Sarwar, & Narayanan, K. M. (1993). Effect of stage of lactation on oligosaccharides level in milk. *Indian Journal of Dairy & Biosciences*, 4, 58-60.

Belitz, H.-D., Grosch, W., & Schieberle, P. (2008). *Lehrbuch der Lebensmittelchemie* (6th ed.). Berlin Heidelberg: Springer.

Berekoven, L., Eckert, W., Ellenrieder, P. (2009). Marktforschung: *Methodische Grundlagen und praktische Anwendung* (12th ed.). Wiesbaden: Gabler.

Bernstein, C. N., Fried, M., Krabshuis, J. H., Cohen, H., Eliakim, R., Fedail, S., ... & Watermeyer, G. (2010). World Gastroenterology Organization Practice Guidelines for the diagnosis and management of IBD in 2010. *Inflammatory Bowel Diseases*, 16(1), 112-124.

Biesiekierski, J. R., Rosella, O., Rose, R., Liels, K., Barrett, J. S., Shepherd, S. J., ... & Muir, J. G. (2011). Quantification of fructans, galacto-oligosacharides and other short-chain carbohydrates in processed grains and cereals. *Journal of Human Nutrition and Dietetics*, 24(2), 154-176.

Binnendijk, K. H., & Rijkers, G. T. (2013). What is a health benefit? An evaluation of EFSA opinions on health benefits with reference to probiotics. *Beneficial Microbes*, 4(3), 223-230.

Blumenthal, M. (1998). *The Complete German Commission E Monographs; Therapeutic Guide to Herbal Medicine*. Boston, MA: Integrative Medicine Communications.

Boehm, G., & Stahl, B. (2007). Oligosaccharides from milk. *The Journal of Nutrition*, 137(3), 847S-849S.

Bowden, P. (2011). *Telling It Like It Is*. Paul Bowden.

Briançon, S., Boini, S., Bertrais, S., Guillemin, F., Galan, P., & Hercberg, S. (2011). Long-term antioxidant supplementation has no effect on health-related quality of life: The randomized, double-blind, placebo-controlled, primary prevention SU.VI.MAX trial. *International Journal of Epidemiology*, 40(6), 1605-1616.

Campbell, J. M., Fahey, G. C., & Wolf, B. W. (1997). Selected indigestible oligosaccharides affect large bowel mass, cecal and fecal short-chain fatty acids, pH and microflora in rats. *The Journal of Nutrition*, 127(1), 130-136.

Chi, W. J., Chang, Y. K., & Hong, S. K. (2012). Agar degradation by microorganisms and agar-degrading enzymes. *Applied Microbiology and Biotechnology*, 94(4), 917-930.

Choi, Y. K; Johlin Jr., F. C.; Summers, R.W., Jackson, M., & Rao, S. S. C. (2003). Fruktose intolerance: an under-recognized problem. *The American Journal of Gastroenterology*, 98(6) 2003, S. 1348-1353.

CIAA (n. d.). *CIAA agreed reference values for GDAs* [Table]. Retrieved from http://gda.fooddrinkeurope.eu/asp2/gdas_portions_rationale.asp?doc_id=127.

Connor, W. E. (2000). Importance of n− 3 fatty acids in health and disease. *The American Journal of Clinical nutrition*, 71(1), 171S-175S.

Coraggio, L. (1990). *Deleterious Effects of Intermittent Interruptions on the Task Performance of Knowledge Workers: A Laboratory Investigation* (Doctoral Dissertation). Retrieved from http://arizona.openrepository.com.

Corazza, G. R., Strocchi, A., Rossi, R., Sirola, D., & Fasbarrini, G. (1988). Sorbitol malabsorption in normal volunteers and in patients with celiac disease. *Gut*, 29(1), 44-48.

Cummings, J. H. (1981). Short chain fatty acids in the human colon. *Gut*, 22(9), 763-779.

Cummings, J. H., & Macfarlane, G. T. (1997). Role of intestinal bacteria in nutrient metabolism. *Journal of Parental and Enteral Nutrition*, 21(6), 357-365.

DGE (2013). Vollwertig essen und trinken nach den 10 Regeln der DGE. 9th Edition, Bonn.

Donker, G. A., Foets, M., & Spreeuwenberg, P. (1999). Patients with irritable bowel syndrome: health status and use of healthcare services. *British Journal of General Practice*, 49(447), 787-792.

Drossman, D. A., Li, Z., Andruzzi, E., Temple, R. D., Talley, N. J., Thompson, W. G. ...Corazziari, E. et al. (1993). US householder survey of functional gastrointestinal disorders: prevalence, sociodemography, and health impact. *Digestive Diseases and Sciences*, 38(9), 1569-1580.

Dukas, L., Willett, W. C., & Giovannucci, E. L. (2003). Association between physical activity, fiber intake, and other lifestyle variables and constipation in a study of women. *The American Journal of Gastroenterology*, 98(8), 1790-1796.

EFSA (2007). Opinion of the scientific panel on dietetic products, nutrition and allergies on a request from the commission related to a notification from epa on lactitol pursuant to article 6, paragraph 11 of directive 2000/13/ec- for permanent exemption from labeling. *The EFSA Journal*, 5(10), 565-570.

EFSA (2012a). Scientific opinion on dietary reference values for protein. *The EFSA Journal*, 10(2), 2557-2622.

EFSA (2012b). Scientific opinion on the substantiation of health claims related to lactobacillus casei dg cncm i-1572 and decreasing potentially pathogenic gastro-intestinal microorganisms (id 2949, 3061, further assessment) pursuant to article 13(1) of regulation (ec) no 1924/2006. *The EFSA Journal*, 10(6), 2723-2637.

EFSA (2012c). Scientific opinion on the tolerable upper intake level of eicosapentaenoic acid (epa), docosahexaenoic acid (dha) and docosapentaenoic acid (dpa). *The EFSA Journal*, 10(7), 2815-2862.

EFSA (2013). scientific opinion on the substantiation of a health claim related to bimuno® gos and reducing gastro-intestinal discomfort pursuant to article 13(5) of regulation (ec) no 1924/2006. *The EFSA Journal*, 11(6), 3259-3268.

Eisenführ, F., Weber, M., & Langer, T. (2010): *Rational Decision Making*, Heidelberg, Berlin: Springer.

Erdman, K., Tunnicliffe, J., Lun, V. M., & Reimer, R. A. (2013). Eating patterns and composition of meals and snacks in elite canadian athletes. *International Journal Of Sport Nutrition & Exercise Metabolism*, 23(3), 210-219.

Evans, J. M., McMahon, A. D., Murray, F. E., McDevitt, D. G., & MacDonald, T. M. (1997). Non-steroidal anti-inflammatory drugs are associated with emergency admission to hospital for colitis due to inflammatory bowel disease. *Gut*, 40(5), 619-622.

Falony, G., Verschaeren, A. De Bruycker, F., De Preter, V., Verbecke, F. L., & De Vuyst L. (2009b). In vitro kinetics of prebiotic inulin-type fructan fermentation by butyrate-producing colon bacteria: implementation of online gas chromatography for quantitative analysis of carbon dioxide and hydrogen gas production. *Applied Environmental Microbiology*, 75(18), 5884-5892.

FAO (2008). Fats and fatty acids in human nutrition. *FAO Food and Nutrition Paper*, 91, 9-20.

Farquhar, P. H., & Keller, L. R. (1989). Preference intensity measurement. *Annals of Operations Research*, 19(1), 205-217.

Farshchi, H. R., Taylor, M. A., & Macdonald, I. A. (2004). Regular meal frequency creates more appropriate insulin sensitivity and lipid profiles compared with irregular meal frequency in healthy lean women. *European Journal of Clinical Nutrition*, 58(7), 1071-1077.

Fasano, A., & Catassi, C. (2001). Current approaches to diagnosis and treatment of celiac disease: an evolving spectrum. *Gastroenterology*, 120(3), 636-651.

Fass, R., Fullerton, S., Naliboff, B., Hirsh, T., & Mayer, E. A. (1998). Sexual dysfunction in patients with irritable bowel syndrom and non-ulcer dyspepsia. *Digestion*, 59(1), 79-85.

Fernández-Bañares, F., Esteve-Pardo, M., de Leon, R., Humbert, P., Cabré, E., Llovet, J. M., & Gassull, M. A. (1993). Sugar malabsorption in functional bowel disease: clinical implications. *American Journal of Gastroenterology*, 88(12), 2044-2050.

Fox, K. (2013). N. t.. In Wells, V., Wyness, L., & Coe, S. (Eds.). The British Nutrition Foundation's 45th anniversary conference: behaviour change in relation to healthier lifestyles. *Nutrition Bulletin*, 38(1), 100-107.

Gaby, A. R. (2005). Adverse effects of dietary fruktose. *Alternative medicine review*, 10(4).

Gay-Crosier, F., Schreiber, G., & Hauser, C. (2000). Anaphylaxis from inulin in vegetables and processed food. *The New England Journal of Medicine*, 342(18), 1372.

German, J., Freeman, S., Lebrilla, C., & Mills, D. (2008). Human milk oligosaccharides: evolution, structures and bioselectivity as substrates for intestinal bacteria, *Nestlé Nutrition Workshop, Pediatric Program*, 62, 205-222.

Gibson, P. R., Newnham, E., Barrett, J. S., Shepherd, S. J., & Muir, J. G. (2007). Review article: Fruktose malabsorption and the bigger picture. *Alimentary Pharmacology & Therapeutics*, 25(4), 349-363.

Gibson, P. R., & Shepherd, S. J. (2010). Evidence-based dietary management of functional gastrointestinal symptoms: the fodmap approach. *Journal of Gastroenterology and Hepatology*, 25(2), 252-258.

Gilbert, P. (2013). N. t.. In Wells, V., Wyness, L., & Coe, S. (Eds.). The British Nutrition Foundation's 45th anniversary conference: behaviour change in relation to healthier lifestyles. *Nutrition Bulletin*, 38(1), 100-107.

Goldstein, R., Braverman, D., & Stankiewicz, H. (2000). Carbohydrate malabsorption and the effect of dietary restriction on symptoms of irritable bowel syndrome and functional bowel complaints. *Israel Medical Association Journal*, 2(8), 583-587.

Gralnek, I. M., Hays, R. D., Kilbourne, A., Naliboff, B., & Mayer, E. A. (2000). The impact of irritable bowel syndrome on health-related quality of life. *Gastroenterology*, 119(3), 654-660.

Hahn, B. A., Kirchdoerfer, L. J., Fullerton, S., & Mayer, S. (1997). Patient perceived severity of irritable bowel syndrome in relation to symptoms, health resource utilization and quality of life. *Alimentary Pharmacology and Therapeutics*, 11(3), 553-559.

Hallert, C., Grant, C., Grehn, S., Grännö, C., Hultén, S., Midhagen, G., ... & Valdimarsson, T. (2002). Evidence of poor vitamin status in coeliac patients on a gluten-free diet for 10 years. *Alimentary Pharmacology & Therapeutics*, 16(7), 1333-1339.

Hanauer, S. B. (2006). Inflammatory bowel disease: epidemiology, pathogenesis, and therapeutic opportunities. *Inflammatory Bowel Diseases*, 12(5), S3-S9.

Hawthorne, B., Lambert, S., Scott, D., & Scott, B. (1991). Food intolerance and the irritable bowel syndrome. *Journal of Human Nutrition and Dietetics*, 4(1), 19–23.

Hawking, S. (n. d.). *Publications*. Retrieved from http://hawking.org.uk/publications.html.

Hillson, M. (2013). N. t.. In Wells, V., Wyness, L., & Coe, S. (Eds.). The British Nutrition Foundation's 45th anniversary conference: behaviour change in relation to healthier lifestyles. *Nutrition Bulletin*, 38(1), 100-107.

Hoekstra, J. H., van Kempen, A. A. M. W., & Kneepkens, C. M. F. (1993). Apple juice malabsorption: fruktose or sorbitol?. *Journal of Pediatric Gastroenterology and Nutrition*, 16(1), 39-42.

Huether, G. (Lecturer) (2014). *Interview mit Prof. Dr. Gerald Hüther zu Angst & Berufung*. Retrieved from http://www.coach-your-self.tv/Startseite/TV/InterviewmitProfDrH%c3%BCtherzuAngstBerufung/tabid/1341/Default.aspx

Hyams, J. S. (1983). Sorbitol intolerance: an unappreciated cause of functional gastrointestinal complaints. *Gastroenterology*, 84(1)1, 30-33.

Hyams, J. S., Etienne, N. L., Leichtner, A. M., & Theuer, R. C. (1988). Carbohydrate malabsorption following fruit juice ingestion in young children. *Pediatrics*, 82(1), 64-68.

Itzkowitz, S. H. & Daniel, H. (2005). Concensus Coference: colorectal cancer screening and surveillance in inflammatory bowel disease. *Inflammatory Bowel Disease*, 11(3).

Jameson, S. (2000). Coeliac disease, insulin-like growth factor, bone mineral density, and zinc. *Scandinavian Journal of Gastroenterology*, 35(8), 894-896.

Jemal, A., Siegel, R., Ward, E., Murray, T., Xu, J. Smigal, C., & Thun, M. J. (2006). Cancer statistics, 2006. *CA: A Cancer Journal for Clinicians*, 56(2), 106-130.

Jensen, R. G., Blanc, B., & Patton, S. (1995). Particulate constituents in human and bovine milks. In Jensen, R. G. (Ed.), *Handbook of Milk Composition* (pp. 51-62). San Diego: Academic Press.

Kennedy, E. (2004). Dietary diversity, diet quality, and body weight regulation. *Nutrition Reviews*, 62(s2), S78-S81.

Kneepkens, C. M. F., Vonk, R. J., & Fernandes, J. (1984). Incomplete intestinal absorption of fruktose. *Archives of Disease in Childhood*, 59(8), 735-738.

Kneepkens, C. M. F., Jakobs, C., & Douwes, A. C. (1989): Apple juice, fruktose, and chronic nonspecific diarrhoea. *Pediatrics*, 148(6), 571-573.

Knudsen, B. K., & Hessov, I. (1995). Recovery of inulin from Jerusalem artichoke (Helianthus tuberosus L.) in the small intestine of man. *British Journal of Nutrition*, 74(01), 101-113.

Komericki, P., Akkilic-Materna, M., Strimitzer, T., Weyermair, K., Hammer, H. F., & Aberer, W. (2012). Oral xylose isomerase decreases breath hydrogen excretion and improves gastrointestinal symptoms in fructose malabsorption – a double-blind, placebo-controlled study. *Alimentary Pharmacology & Therapeutics*, 36(10), 980-987.

Kornbluth, A., & Sachar, D. B. (2004). Ulcerative colitis practice guidelines in adults (update): American College of Gastroenterology, Practice Parameters Committee. *The American Journal of Gastroenterology*, 99(7), 1371-1385.

Kuhn, R., & Gauhe, A. (1965). Bestimmung der bindungsstelle von sialinsäureresten in oligosacchariden mit hilfe von perjodat. *Chemische Berichte*, 98(2), 395-314.

Kupper, C. (2005). Dietary guidelines and implementation for celiac disease. *Gastroenterology*, 128(4), 121-127.

Kushi, L. H., Doyle, C., McCullough, M., Rock, C. L., Demark-Wahnefried, W. Bandera, E. V., ... & Gansler, T. (2012). American cancer society guidelines on nutrition and physical activity for cancer prevention. *CA: A Cancer Journal for Clinicians*, 62(1), 30-67.

Ladas, S. D., Grammenos, I., Tassios, P. S., & Raptis, S. A. (2000). Coincidental malabsorption of laktose, fruktose, and sorbitol ingested at low doses is not Common in normal adults. *Digestive Diseases and Sciences*, 45(12), 2357-2362.

Langkilde, A. M., Andersson, H., Schweizer, T. F., & Würsch, P. (1994). Digestion and absorption of sorbitol, maltitol and isomalt from the small bowel. A study in ileostomy subjects. *European Journal of Clinical Nutrition*, 48(11), 768-775.

Latulippe, M. E., & Skoog, S. M. (2011). Fruktose malabsorption and intolerance: effects of fruktose with and without simultaneous glucose ingestion. *critical Reviews in Food Science and Nutrition*, 51(7), 583-592.

Le, A. S., & Mulderrig, K. B. (2001). *Sorbitol and Mannitol*. Nabors, O'B. (Ed.). New York, NY: Marcel Dekker.

Ledochowski, M., Sperner-Unterweger, B., Widner, B., & Fuchs, D. (1998a). Fruktose malabsorption is associated with early signs of mentral depression. *European Journal of Medical Research*, 3(6), 295-298.

Ledochowski, M., Sperner-Unterweger, B., & Fuchs, D. (1998b). Laktose malabsorption is associated with early signs of mental depression in females – a preliminary report. *Digestive Diseases and Sciences*, 43(11), 2513-2517.

Ledochowski, M., Überall, F., Propst, T., & Fuchs, D. (1999). Fruktose malabsorption is associated with lower plasma folic acid concentrations in middle-aged subjects. *Clinical Chemistry*, 45(11), 2013-2014.

Ledochowski, M., Widner, B., Bair, H., Probst, T., & Fuchs, D. (2000a). Fruktose-and sorbitol-reduced diet improves mood and gastrointestinal disturbances in fruktose malabsorbers. *Scandinavian Journal of Gastroenterology*, 35(10), 1048-1052.

Ledochowski, M., Widner, B., Sperner-Unterweger, B., Probst, T., Vogel, W., & Fuchs, D. (2000b). Carbohydrate malabsobtion syndromes and early signs of mental depression in females. *Digestive Diseases and Sciences*, 45(12), 1255-1259. [Anm. d. Verf.: Die Studie ist für Männer nicht aussagekräftig, da die Stichprobengröße zu klein ist.]

Leinoel (n. d.). *Leinöl(Leinsamen)*. Retrieved from http://www.vitalstoff-journal.de/vitalstoff-lexikon/l/leinoel-leinsamen.

Lewis, S. J., & Heaton, K. W. (1997). Stool form scale as a useful guide to intestinal transit time. *Scandinavian Journal of Gastroenterology*, 32(9), 920-924.

Lifschitz, C. H. (2000). Carbohydrate absorption from fruit juices in infants. *Pediatrics*, 105(1), e4.

Lombardi, D. A., Jin, K., Courtney, T. K., Arlinghaus, A., Folkard, S., Liang, Y., & Perry, M. J. (2014). The effects of rest breaks, work shift start time, and sleep on the onset of severe injury among workers in the People's Republic of China. *Scandinavian Journal of Work, Environment & Health*, 40(2), 146-155.

Lomer, M. C. E., Parkes, G. C., & Sanderson, J. D. (2008). Review article: Laktose intolerance in clinical practice – myths and realities. *Alimentary Pharmacology & Therapeutics*, 27(2), 93-103.

Longstreth, G. F., Thompson, W. G., chey, W. D., Houghton, L. A., Mearin, F., & Spiller, R. C. (2006). Functional bowel disorders. *Gastroenterology*, 130(5), 1480-1491.

Maintz, L., & Novak, N. (2007). Histamine and histamine intolerance. *The American Journal of Clinical Nutrition*, 85(5), 1185-1196.

Makras, L., Van Acker, G., & De Vuyst, L. (2005). Lactobacillus paracasei subsp. paracasei 8700: 2 degrades inulin-type fructans exhibiting different degrees of polymerization. *Applied and Environmental Microbiology*, 71(11), 6531-6537.

Mccoubrey, H., Parkes, G. C., Sanderson, J. D., & Lomer, M. C. E. (2008). Nutritional intakes in irritable bowel syndrome. *Journal of Human Nutrition and Dietetics*, 21(4), 396-397.

McKenzie, Y. A., Alder, A., Anderson, W. Goddard, L, Gulia, P., Jankovich, E. …Lomer, M. C. E. (2012). British dietic association evidence-based guidelines for the dietary management of irritable bowel syndrome in adults. *Journal of Human Nutrition and Dietics*, 25(3), 260-274.

Meyrand, M., Dallas, D. C., caillat, H., Bouvier, F., Martin, P., & Barile, D. (2013). Comparison of milk oligosaccharides between goats with and without the genetic ability to synthesize αs1-casein. *Small Ruminant Research*, 113(2), 411-420.

Michel, G., Nyval-Collen, P., Barbeyron, T., czjzek, M., & Helbert, W. (2006). Bioconversion of red seaweed galactans: a focus on bacterial agarases and Carrageenases. *Applied Microbiology and Biotechnology*, 71(1), 23-33.

Michie, S. (2013). N. t.. In Wells, V., Wyness, L., & Coe, S. (Eds.). The British Nutrition Foundation's 45th anniversary conference: Behaviour change in relation to healthier lifestyles. *Nutrition Bulletin*, 38(1), 100-107.

Mishkin, D., Sablauskas, L., Yalovsky, M., & Mishkin, S. (1997). Fruktose and sorbitol malabsorption in ambulatory patients with functional dyspepsia: comparison with laktose maldigestion/malabsorption. *Digestive Diseases and Sciences*, 42(12), 2591-2598.

Molodecky N. A., Soon, I. S., Rabi, D. M., et al. (2012). Increasing incidence and precalence of the inflammatory bowel diseases with time, based on systematic review. *Gastroenterology*, 142(1), 46-54.

Monash University (2014). *The Monash University Low Foodmap Diet* [Software]. Available from http://www.med.monash.edu/cecs/gastro/fodmap/education.html

Montalto, M., Curigliano, V., Santoro, L., Vastola, M., Cammarota, G., Manna, R., ... & Gasbarrini, G. (2006). Management and treatment of laktose malabsorption. *World Journal of Gastroenterology*, 12(2), 187.

Molis, C., Flourié, B., Ouarne, F., Gailing, M. F., Lartigue, S., Guibert, A., Bornet, F., & Galmiche, F. P. (1996). Digestion, excretion, and energy value of fructooligosaccharides in healthy humans. *The American Society for Clinical Nutrition*, 64(3), 324-328.

Mosby's Medical Dictionary (8th ed.). St. Louis, MO: Mosby.

Moshfegh, A. J., James, E. F., Goldman, J. P., & Ahuja, J. L. C. (1999). Presence of inulin and oligofruktose in the diets of Americans. *The Journal of Nutrition*, 129(7), 1407S-1411S.

Mount Sinai (n. d.). *Fiber Chart*. Retrieved from https://www.wehealny.org/healthinfo/dietaryfiber/fibercontentchart.html.

Mozaffarian, D., & Wu, J. H. (2011). Omega-3 fatty acids and cardiovascular disease effects on risk factors, molecular pathways, and clinical events. *Journal of the American College of Cardiology*, 58(20), 2047-2067.

Muir, J. G., Shepherd, S. J., Rosella, O., Rose, R., Barrett, J. S., & Gibson, P. R. (2007). Fructan and free fruktose content of common Australian vegetables and fruit. *Journal of Agricultural and Food Chemistry*, 55(16), 6619-6627.

Muir, J. G., Rose, R., Rosella, O., Liels, K., Barrett, J. S., Shepherd, S. J., & Gibson, P. R. (2009). Measurement of short-chain carbohydrates in common Australian vegetables and fruits by high-performance liquid chromatography (HPLC). *Journal of Agricultural and Food Chemistry*, 57(2), 554-565.

Nanda, R., James, R., Smith, H., Dudley, C. R. K., & Jewell, D. P. (1989). Food intolerance and the irritable bowel syndrome. *Gut*, 30(8), 1099-1104.

National Digestive Diseases Information Clearinghouse (2014). Crohn's disease. *NIH Publication*, 14-3410.

National Digestive Diseases Information Clearinghouse (2014). Diverticular disease. *NIH Publication*, 13-1163.

National Digestive Diseases Information Clearinghouse (2014). Ulcerative colitis. *NIH Publication*, 14-1597.

Necas, J., Bartosikova, L. (2013). Carageenan: a review. *Veterinarni Medicina*, 58(4), 187-205.

Nelis, G. F., Vermeeren, M. A., & Jansen, W. (1990). Role of fruktose-sorbitol malabsorbtion in the irritable bowel syndrome. *Gastroenterology*, 99(4), 1016-1020.

Newburg, D. S. & Neubauer, S. H. (1995). Carbohydrates in milks: analysis, quantities, and significance. In Jensen, R. G. (Ed.), *Handbook of Milk Composition* (pp. 273-349). San Diego: Academic Press.

NICNAS (2008). Multiple chemical sensitivity: identifying key research needs. *Scientific Review Report*.

Nucera, G., Gabrielli, M., Lupascu, A., Lauritano, E. C., Santoliquido, A., cremonini, F., ...Gasbarrini, A. (2005). Abnormal breath tests to laktose, fruktose and sorbitol in irritable bowel syndrome may be explained by small intestinal bacterial overgrowth. *Alimentary Pharmacology & Therapeutics*, 21(11), 1391-1395.

O'Connell, J. B., Maggard, M. A., & Ko, C. Y. (2004). Colon cancer survival rates with the new American Joint Committee on Cancer sixth edition staging. *Journal of the National Cancer Institute*, 96(19), 1420-1425.

O'Connell, S., & Walsh, G. (2006). Physicochemical characteristics of commercial lactases relevant to their application in the alleviation of laktose intolerance. *Applied Biochemistry and Biotechnology*, 134(2), 179-191.

Ong, D., Mitchell, S., Barrett, J., Shepherd, S., Irving, P., Biesiekierski, J., & ... Muir, J. (2010). Manipulation of dietary short chain carbohydrates alters the pattern of gas production and genesis of symptoms in irritable bowel syndrome. *Journal of Gastroenterology & Hepatology*, 25(8), 1366-1373.

Park, Y. K., & Yetley, E. A. (1993). Intakes and food sources of fruktose in the United States. *The American Journal of Clinical Nutrition*, 58(5), 737S-747S.

Parker, T. J., Naylor, S. J., Riordan, A. M., & Hunter, J. O. (1995). Management of patients with food intolerance in irritable bowel syndrome. The development and use of an exclusion diet. *Journal of Human Nutrition and Dietetics*, 8(3), 159-166.

Peery, A. F., Barrett, P. R. Park, D., et al. (2012). A high-fiber diet does not protect against asymptomatic diverticulosis. *Gastroenterology*, 142(2), 266-272.

Petitpierre, M., Gumowski, P., & Girard, J. P. (1985). Irritable bowel syndrome and hypersensitivity to food. *Annals of Allergy, Asthma & Immunology*, 54(6), 538-540.

Quigley, E., Fried, M., Gwee, K. A., Olano, C., Guarner, F., Khalif, I., ... & Le Mair, A. W. (2009). Irritable bowel syndrome: a global perspective. *WGO Practice Guideline*.

Quigley, E., M., M., Hunt, R. H., Emmanuel, A., & Hungin, A. P. S. (2013). *Irritable bowel syndrome (ibs): what is it, what causes it and can i do anything about it?* Retrieved from http://client.blueskybroadcastcom/WGO/ index.html.

Raithel, M., Weidenhiller, M., Hagel, A.-F.-K., Hetterich, U., Neurath, M. F., & Konturek, P. C. (2013). The malabsorption of commonly occurring mono and disaccharides: levels of investigation and differential diagnoses. *Dtsch Arztebl Int,* 110(46), 775-782.

Rex, D. K., Johnson, D. A., Anderson, J. C., Schoenfeld, P. S., Burke, C. A., & Inadomi, J. M. (2009). American College of Gastroenterology guidelines for colorectal cancer screening 2008. *The American Journal of Gastroenterology,* 104(3), 739-750.

Riby, J. E., Fujisawa, T., & Kretchmer, N. (1993). Fruktose absorption. *The American Journal of Clinical Nutrition,* 58(5), 748S-753S.

Ross, A. C., Manson, J. E., Abrams, S. A., Aloia, J. F., Brannon, P. M., Clinton, S. K., ... & Shapses, S. A. (2011). The 2011 report on dietary reference intakes for calcium and vitamin D from the Institute of Medicine: what clinicians need to know. *Journal of Clinical Endocrinology & Metabolism,* 96(1), 53-58.

Rubio-Tapia, A., Hill, I. D., Kelly, C. P., Calderwood, A. H., & Murray, J. A. (2013). ACG clinical guidelines: diagnosis and management of celiac disease.*The American Journal of Gastroenterology,* 108(5), 656-676.

Rumessen, J. J., & Gudmand-Høyer, E. (1986). Absorption capacity of fruktose in healthy adults. comparison with sucrose and its constituent monosaccharides. *Gut,* 27(10), 1161-1168.

Rumessen, J. J., & Gudmand-Høyer, E. (1987). Malabsoption of fruktose-sorbitol mixtures. Interactions causing abdominal distress. *Scandinavian Journal of Gastroenterology,* 22(4), 431-436.

Rumessen, J. J. (1992). Fruktose and related food carbohydrates. sources, intake, absorbtion, and clinical implications. *Scandinavian Journal of Gastroenterology,* 27(10), 819-828.

Ruppin, H., Bar-Meir, S., Soergel, K. H., Wood, C. M., & Schmitt Jr, M. G. (1980). Absorption of short-chain fatty acids by the colon. *Gastroenterology,* 78(6), 1500-1507.

Rycroft, C. E., Jones, M. R., Gibson, G. R., & Rastall, R. A. (2001). A comparative in vitro evaluation of the fermentation properties of prebiotic oligosaccharides. *Journal of Applied Microbiology,* 91(5), 878-887.

Scientific Community on Food (2000*). Opinion of the Scientific Committee on Food on the tolerable upper intake level of folate.* Retrieved from: www.ec.europa.eu/food/fc/sc/scf/out80e_en.pdf

Shepherd, S. J., & Gibson, P. R. (2006). Fruktose malabsorption and symptoms of irritable bowel syndrome: guidelines for effective dietary management. *Journal of the American Dietetic Association*, 106(10), 1631-1639.

Shepherd, S. J., Parker, F. C., Muir, J. G., & Gibson, P. R. (2008). Dietary triggers of abdominal symptoms in patients with irritable bowel syndrome: randomized placebo-controlled evidence. *Clinical Gastroenterology and Hepatology*, 6(7), 765-771.

Silk, D. B. A., Davis, A., Vulevic, J., Tzortzis, G., & Gibson, G. R. (2009). Clinical trial: the effects of a trans-galactooligosaccharide prebiotic on faecal microbiota and symptoms in irritable bowel syndrome. *Alimentary Pharmacology & Therapeutics*, 29(5), 508-518.

Simopoulos, A. P. (1999). Essential fatty acids in health and chronic disease. *The American Journal of Clinical Nutrition*, 70(3), 560s-569s.

Speier, C., Vessey, I., & Valacich, J. S. (2003). The effects of interruptions, task complexity, and information presentation on computer-supported decision-making performance. *Decision Sciences*, 34(4), 771-797.

Stefanini, G. F., Saggioro, A., Alvisi, V., Angelini, G., capurso, L., Di, L. G., ...Melzi, G. (1995). Oral cromolyn sodium in comparison with elimination diet in the irritable bowel syndrome, diarrheic type. multicenter study of 428 patients. *Scandinavian Journal of Gastroenterology*, 30(6), 535–541.

Stockwell, M. (n. d.). *Awards/Events*. Retrieved from www.melissastockwell.com/Melissa_Stockwell/Awards.html.

Stubbs, J. (2013). N. t.. In Wells, V., Wyness, L., & Coe, S. (Eds.). The British Nutrition Foundation's 45th anniversary conference: behaviour change in relation to healthier lifestyles. *Nutrition Bulletin*, 38(1), 100-107.

Suarez, F. L., Savaiano, D. A., & Levitt, M. D. (1995). A comparison of symptoms after the consumption of milk or lactose-hydrolyzed milk by people with self-reported severe lactose intolerance. *New England Journal of Medicine*, 333(1), 1-4.

Suarez, F. L., Springfield, J., Furne, J. K., Lohrmann, T. T., Kerr, P. S., & Levitt, M. D. (1999). Gas production in humans ingesting a soybean flour derived from beans naturally low in oligosaccharides. *The American Journal of Clinical Nutrition*, 69(1), 135-139.

Sundhedsstyrelsen og Fødevareministeriet (2009). *Cøliaki og mad uden Gluten* (4th ed.). København: Sundhedsstyrelsen.

Tarpila, S., Tarpila, A., Grohn, P., Silvennoinen, T., & Lindberg, L. (2004). Efficacy of ground flaxseed on constipation in patients with irritable bowel syndrome. *Current Topics in Nutraceutical Research*, 2(2), 119–125.

Test (2008). Schneller, schöner, stärker. *test – Journal Gesundheit*, 43(02), 88-92.

Teuri, U., Vapaatalo, H., & Korpela, R. (1999). Fructooligosaccharides and lactulose cause more symptoms in laktose maldigesters and subjects with pseudohypolactasia than in control laktose digesters. *The American Journal of Clinical Nutrition*, 69(5), 973-979.

Thompson, Kyle (2006). *Bristol Stool Chart* [Graphical illustration]. Retrieved from http://commons.wikimedia.org/wiki/File:Bristol_Stool_chart.png

Nanda, R., Shu, L. H., & Thomas, J. R. (2012). A fodmap diet update: craze or credible. *Practical Gastroenterology*, 10(12), 37-46.

Toschke, A. M., Thorsteinsdottir, K. H., & von Kries, R. (2009). Meal frequency, breakfast consumption and childhood obesity. *International Journal of Pediatric Obesity*, 4(4), 242-248.

Tou, J. C., Chen, J., & Thompson, L. U. (1998). Flaxseed and its lignan precursor, secoisolariciresinol diglycoside, affect pregnancy outcome and reproductive development in rats. *The Journal of Nutrition*, 128(11), 1861-1868.

Truswell, A. S., Seach, J. M., & Thorburn, A. W. (1988). Incomplete absorption of pure fruktose in healthy subjects and the facilitating effect of glucose. *The American Journal of Clinical Nutrition*, 48(6), 1424-1430.

U. S. Department of Agriculture and U. S. Department of Health and Human Services (2010). *Dietary Guidelines for Americans* (7th ed.). Washington, Dc: U. S. Government Printing Office.

U. S. Department of Agriculture, Agricultural Research Service (2013). *USDA National Nutrient Database for Standard Reference*, Release 26. Retrieved from: http://www.ars.usda.gov/ba/bhnrc /ndl.

van Loo, J., Coussement, P., De Leenheer, L., Hoebregs, H., & Smits, G. (1995). On the presence of inulin and oligofruktose as natural ingredients in the western diet. *Critical Reviews in Food Science and Nutrition*, 35(6), 525–552.

Varea, V., de Carpi, J. M., Puig, C., Alda, J. A., camacho, E., Ormazabal, A., ... & Gómez, L. (2005). Malabsorption of carbohydrates and depression in Children and adolescents. *Journal of Pediatric Gastroenterology and Nutrition*, 40(5), 561-565.

Verhoef, P., Stampfer, M. J., Buring, J. F., Gaziano, J. M., Allen, R. H., Stabler, S. P., ... & Willett, W. C. (1996). Homocysteine metabolism and risk of myocardial infarction: relation with vitamins B6, B12, and folate. *American Journal of Epidemiology*, 143(9), 845-859.

Vernia, P., Ricciardi, M. R., Frandina, C., Bilotta, T., & Frieri, G. (1995). laktose malabsorption and irritable bowel syndrome. Effect of a long-term laktose-free diet. *The Italian Journal of Gastroenterology*, 27(3), 117-121.

Vesa, T. H., Korpela, R. A., & Sahi, T. (1996). Tolerance to small amounts of laktose in laktose maldigesters. *The AmericanJournal of Clinical Nutrition*, 64(2), 197-20.

Virtanen, S. M., Räsänen, L., Mäenpää, J., & Åkerblom, H. K. (1987). Dietary survey of Finnish adolescent diabetics and non-diabetic controls. *Acta Paediatrica*, 76(5), 801-808.

Vos, M. B., Kimmons, J. E., Gillespie, C., Welsh, J., & Blanck, H. M. (2008). Dietary fruktose consumption among US children and adults: the third National Health and Nutrition Examination Survey. *The Medscape Journal of Medicine*, 10(7), 160.

Watson, B. D. (2008). Public health and carrageenan regulation : a review and analysis. *Journal of Applied Phycology*, 20(5), 505-513.

Webb, F. S., & Whitney, E. N. (2008). *Nutrition: Concepts and Controversies* (11th ed.). Belmont, CA: Thomson/ Wadsworth.

Wedlake, L., Slack, N., Andreyev, H. J. N., & Whelan, K. (2014). Fiber in the treatment and maintenance of inflammatory bowel disease: a systematic review of randomized controlled trials. *Inflammatory bowel diseases*, 20(3), 576-586.

Welch, C. E., Allen, A. W., & Donaldons, G. A. (1953). An appraisal of resection of the colon for diverticulitis of the sigmoid. *Annals of Surgery*, 138(3), 332-343.

Wells, N. E. J., Hahn, B. A., & Whorwell, P. J. (1997). Clinical economics review: irritable bowel syndrome. *Allimentary Pharmacology and Therapeutics*, 11, 1019-1030.

—

Sources regarding the prevalence of IBS:
USA
Longstreth, G. F., & Wolde-Tsadik, G. (1993). Irritable bowel-type symptoms in hmo examinees. *Digestive Diseases and Sciences*, 38(9), 1581-1589.

Talley, N. J., Zinsmeister, A. R., van Dyke, C., & Melton, L. J. (1991). Epidemiology of colonic symptoms and the irritable bowel syndrome. *Gastroenterology*, 101(4), 927-934.

O'Keefe, E. A., Talley, N. J., Zinsmeister, A. R., & Jacobsen, S. J. (1995). Bowel disorders impair functional status and quality of life in the elerdly: a population-based study. *Journal of Gastroenterology*, 50A, M184-M189.

Great Britain
Jones, R., & Lydeard, S. (1992). Irritable bowel syndrom in the general population. *British Medical Journal*, 304(6819), 87-90.

Japan and the Netherlands
  Schlemper, R. J., van der Werf, S. D. J., Vandenbroucke, J. P., Blemond, I., & Lamers, C. B. H. W. (1993). Peptic ulcer, non-ulcer dysepsia and irritable bowel syndrom in the Netherlands and Japan. *Scandinavian Journal of Gastroenterology*, 28(200), 33-41.
Nigeria
  Olubuykle, I. O., Olawuyl, F., & Fasanmade, A. A. (1995). A study of irritable bowel syndrom diagnosed by manning Criteria in an African population. *Digestive Diseases and Sciences*, 40(5), 983-985.

—

  Wilder-Smith, C. H., Materna, A., Wermelinger, C., & Schuler, J. (2013). Fruktose and laktose intolerance and malabsorption testing: the relationship with symptoms in functional gastrointestinal disorders. *Alimentary Pharmacology and Therapeutics*, 37(11), 1074-1083.
  Winterfeldt, D. von, & Edwards, W. (1986). *Decision Analysis and Behavioral Research*. Cambridge: Cambridge University Press.
  Wittstock, A. (1949). *Marc Aurel – Selbstbetrachtungen*. Stuttgart: Reclam.
  Zohar, D. (1999). When things go wrong: The effect of daily work hassles on effort, exertion and negative mood. *Journal of Occupational and Organizational Psychology*, 72(3), 265-283.

Food Index

A

3 Musketeers® 122
7 UP® 98
9-grain Wheat bread 143
After Eight® Thin Chocolate Mints 122
Ale 85
Alfalfa sprouts 152
All-Bran® Original (Kellogg's®) 103
Almond butter, salted 106
Almond butter, unsalted 106
Almond cookies 117
Almond milk, vanilla or other flavors, unsweetened 236
Almond paste (Marzipan) 122
Almonds, honey roasted 122
Almonds, raw 114
Alpine Lace 25% Reduced Fat, Mozzarella 106
Amaranth Flakes (Arrowhead Mills) 103
Amaretto 85
American cheese 143
American cheese, processed 106
Americano, decaf, without flavored syrup 91
Americano, with flavored syrup 91
Americano, without flavored syrup 91
Apple banana strawberry juice 95
Apple cake, glazed 117
Apple grape juice 95
Apple juice or cider, made from frozen 85
Apple juice or cider, unsweetened 85
Apple strudel 117
Applejack liquor 85
Applesauce, canned, sweetened 147
Applesauce, canned, unsweetened 147
Apricot nectar 95
Apricot, dried, cooked, sweetened 147
Apricot, dried, uncooked 147
Apricot, fresh 147
Aquavit 85
Arby's® macaroni and cheese 127
Arby's® orange juice 95
Archway® Ginger Snaps 117
Archway® Oatmeal Raisin Cookies 117
Archway® Peanut Butter Cookies 117
Artichoke, globe raw 152
Arugula, raw 152
Asian noodle bowl, vegetables only 127
Asparagus, raw 152
Au gratin potato, prepared from fresh 136
Avocado, green skin, Florida type 152

B

Baby food, Gerber Graduates® Organic Pasta Pick-Ups Three Cheese Ravioli 127
Baby food, zwieback 114
bacon 143
Bacon EGG® and Cheese BK Muffin® 138
Baguette 101
Baking powder 162
Bamboo shoots, canned and drained 152
Banana, chips 147
Banana, fresh 147
Barbecue sauce 138
Barley flour 162

Basmati rice, cooked in unsalted water 136
BBQ roasted jalapeno sauce 138
Beef bacon (kosher) 132
Beef steak, chuck, visible fat eaten 132
Beef with noodles soup, condensed 127
Beer 85
Beer, low alcohol 85
Beer, low carb 85
Beer, non alcoholic 85
Beets, raw 152
Ben & Jerry's® Ice Cream, Brownie Batter 159
Ben & Jerry's® Ice Cream, Chocolate Chip Cookie Dough 159
Ben & Jerry's® Ice Cream, Chubby Hubby® 159
Ben & Jerry's® Ice Cream, Chunky Monkey® 159
Ben & Jerry's® Ice Cream, Half Baked 159
Ben & Jerry's® Ice Cream, Karamel Sutra® 159
Ben & Jerry's® Ice Cream, New York Super Fudge Chunk® 159
Ben & Jerry's® Ice Cream, One Sweet Whirled 159
Ben & Jerry's® Ice Cream, Peanut Butter Cup 159
Ben & Jerry's® Ice Cream, Phish Food® 159
Ben & Jerry's® Ice Cream, Vanilla For A Change 159
Biscotti, chocolate, nuts 117
BK Big Fish® 138
BK Fresh Apple Slices 138
Black beans, cooked from dried 152
Black cherry juice 95
Black currant juice 95
Black olives 152
Black Russian 85
Blackberries, fresh 147
Blackberry juice 95
Bloody Mary 85
BLT Salad® with TenderCrisp chicken (no dressing or croutons) 138
Blue cheese 106
Blueberries, fresh 147
Bockwurst 132
Bok choy, raw 152
Bologna, beef ring 106
Bologna, combination of meats, light (reduced fat) 106
Boston Market® 1/4 white rotisserie chicken, with skin 132
Boston Market® macaroni and cheese 127
Boston Market® roasted turkey breast 132
Boston Market® sweet corn 136
Bourbon 85
Boysenberries, fresh 147
Brandy 85
Bratwurst 132
Bratwurst, beef 132
Bratwurst, light (reduced fat) 132
Bratwurst, made with beer 132
Bratwurst, made with beer, cheese-filled 132
Bratwurst, turkey 132
Braunschweiger 132
Brazil nuts, unsalted 114
Breath mint, regular 122
Breath mint, sugar free 122
Breyers® Ice Cream, Natural Vanilla, Lactose Free 159
Breyers® Light! Boosts Immunity Yogurt, all flavors 236
Breyers® No Sugar Added Ice Cream, Vanilla 236
Breyers® YoCrunch Light Nonfat Yogurt, with granola 236

Brie cheese 106
Broccoli flower (green cauliflower), cooked 152
Broccoli, raw 152
Brown mushrooms (Italian or Crimini, raw 152
Brown sugar 122
Brownie, chocolate, fat free 117
Brussels sprouts, cooked from fresh 152
Bulgur, home cooked 136
Burgundy wine, red 86
Burgundy wine, white 86
Butter cracker 117
Butter, light, salted 106
Butter, unsalted 106
Buttermels® (Switzer's®) 122
Butternut squash soup 127

C

Cabbage, green, cooked 153
Cabbage, red, cooked 153
Cabbage, savoy, raw 153
Cabot® Non Fat Yogurt, plain 236
Cabot® Non Fat Yogurt, vanilla 236
Caesar Salad (no dressing or croutons) 138
Caesar salad dressing 140
Cafe au lait, without flavored syrup 91
Cafe latte, flavored syrup 91
Cafe latte, without flavored syrup 91
Calzone, cheese 127
Camembert cheese 106
Camomile tea 91
Campari® 86
Candy necklace 122
Canfield's® Root Beer 98
Canfield's® Root Beer, diet 98
Cantaloupe, fresh 147
Cape Cod 86
Cappuccino, canned 91
Cappuccino, decaf, with flavored syrup 91
Cappuccino, decaf, without flavored syrup 91
Capri Sun®, all flavors 95
Carambola (starfruit), fresh 147
Caramel or sugar coated popcorn, store bought 114
Carrot cake, glazed, homemade 117
Carrot juice 95
Carrots, cooked from fresh 153
Carrots, raw 153
Cascadian Farm® Organic Gran. Bar, Dark Chocolate Cranberry 103
Cashews, raw 114
Casserole (hot dish), with tomato 135
Casserole (hot dish), rice with beef, tomato base, vegetables other than dark green, cheese or gravy 127
Cauliflower, cooked from frozen 153
Caviar 132
Celeriac (celery root), cooked from fresh 153
Celery, cooked 153
Chai tea 91
Chalupas Supreme® with beef, beans, cheese 145
Champagne punch 86
Champagne, white 86
Chard, raw or blanched, marinated in oil 153
Chardonnay 86
Chayote squash, cooked 153
Cheddar cheese 143
Cheddar cheese, natural 106
Cheerios® Snack Mix, all 103
Cheese cracker 114
Cheese gnocchi 136
Cheese sauce, store bought 106
Cheeseburger 138
Cheesecake, plain or flavored, homemade 117
Cherry Coke® 98

Cherry pie, bottom crust only 117
Chestnuts, boiled, steamed 153
Chestnuts, roasted 114
Chewing gum 122
Chewing gum, sugar free 122
Chia seeds 114
Chicken and dumplings soup, condensed 127
Chicken breast, spicy crispy 140
Chicken cake or patty 135
Chicken fricassee with gravy, American style 132
Chicken Littles with sauce 140
Chicken noodle soup with vegetables, can 127
Chicken with cheese sauce, vegetables other than dark green 135
Chicken wonton soup, prepared from condensed can 127
Chicory coffee 91
Chicory coffee powder, unprepared 153
Chicory greens, raw 153
Chili with beans, beef, canned 127
Chipotle southwest salad dressing 143
Chips Ahoy!® Chewy Gooey Caramel Cookies (Nabisco®) 117
Chobani® Nonfat Greek Yogurt, Black Cherry 236
Chobani® Nonfat Greek Yogurt, Lemon 236
Chobani® Nonfat Greek Yogurt, Peach 236
Chobani® Nonfat Greek Yogurt, Raspberry 236
Chobani® Nonfat Greek Yogurt, Strawberry 236
Chocolate cake, glazed, store 117
Chocolate Chex® (General Mills®) 103
Chocolate chip cookie 143
Chocolate chip cookies, store bought 118
Chocolate chunk cookie 143
Chocolate cookies, iced, store bought 118
Chocolate pudding, store bought 236
Chocolate pudding, store bought, no sugar 236
Chocolate sandwich cookies, double filling 118
Chocolate sandwich cookies, sugar free 118
Chocolate truffles 122
Chop suey, chicken 128
Chop suey, tofu, no noodles 128
Cinnamon crispas 118
Cinnamon toast crunch® (General Mills®) 103
Cinnamon Toasters® (Malt-O-Meal®) 103
Clams, with mushroom, onions, & bread 132
Classic Fruit Chocolates (Liberty Orchards®) 122
Clementine, fresh 147
Clif Bar®, Chocolate Chip 83
Clif Bar®, Crunchy Peanut Butter 83
Clif Bar®, Oatmeal Raisin Walnut 83
Club soda 86
Cocoa Krispies® (Kellogg's®) 103
Cocoa Puffs® (General Mills®) 103
Coconut Bars, nuts 122
Coconut cream (liquid from grated meat) 114
Coconut milk, fresh (liquid from grated meat, water added) 114
Coconut, dried, shredded or flaked, unsweetened 114
Coconut, fresh 114
Coffee substitute, prepared 91

Coffee, prepared from flavored mix, no sugar 91
Cognac 86
Cointreau® 86
Coke Zero® 98
Coke® 98
Coke® with Lime 98
Colby Jack cheese 106
Cole slaw 140
Coleslaw, with apples and raisins, mayo dressing 153
Coleslaw, with pineapple, mayo dressing 153
Collards, raw 153
Corn Chex® (General Mills®) 103
Corn Flakes (Kellogg's®) 103
Cornbread, from mix 136
Cornbread, homemade 136
Cottage cheese, 1% fat, lactose reduced 106
Cottage cheese, uncreamed dry curd 236
Couscous, cooked 136

Cracked wheat bread, with raisins 101
Cranberries, dried (Craisins®) 148
Cranberries, fresh 148
Cranberry juice cocktail, with apple juice 95
Cranberry juice cocktail, with blueberry juice 95
Cream cheese spread 107
Cream cheese, whipped, flavored 107
Cream cheese, whipped, plain 107
Cream of asparagus soup, condensed can 128
Cream of broccoli soup, condensed 128
Cream of celery soup, homemade 128
Cream of chicken soup, condensed 128
Cream of mushroom soup, from condensed can 128

Cream of potato soup mix, dry 128
Cream of spinach soup mix, dry 128
Creamed chicken 135
Creamy buffalo sauce 140
Creme de Cocoa 86
Creme de menthe 86
Crepe, plain 118
Crispy Chicken Caesar Salad 140
Crispy Twister without sauce 140
Crispy Twister® with sauce 140
Croissant, chocolate 118
Croissant, fruit 118
Crunchy Nut Roasted Nut & Honey (Kellogg's®) 103
Cucumber, raw, with peel 154
Cucumber, raw, without peel 154
Curacao 86
Currants, fresh, black 148
Currants, fresh, red and white 148

D

Daiquiri 86
Dairy Queen® Foot Long Hot Dog 128
Dandelion tea 92
Danish pastry, frosted, with cheese filling 118
Dannon® Activia® Light Yogurt, vanilla 110
Dannon® Activia® Yogurt, plain 110
Dannon® Greek Yogurt Honey 110
Dannon® Greek Yogurt, Plain 110
Dannon® la Crème Yogurt, fruit flavors 110
Dare Breaktime Ginger Cookies 118
Dare® Lemon Crème Cookies 118
Dark chocolate Bar 50% 122
Dark chocolate Bar 60%-69% cacao 123
Dark chocolate Bar 70%-85% cacao 123

Dark chocolate Bar, sugar free 123
Dark Fruit Chocolates (Liberty Orchards®) 123
Dark Fruit Chocolates, Sugar Free (Liberty Orchards®) 123
Dates 148
Demitasse 92
Diet 7 UP® 98
Diet Coke® 98
Diet Dr. Pepper® 98
Diet Pepsi®, fountain 98
Doritos® Tortilla Chips, Nacho Cheese 114
Doughnut, glazed, coconut topping 118
Doughnut, glazed, plain 118
Doughnut, sugared 118
Dove® Promises, Milk Chocolate 92
Dreyer's® Grand Ice Cream, Chocolate 159
Dreyer's® No Sugar Added Ice Cream, Triple Chocolate 159
Drumstick® (sundae cone) 160

E
Earl Grey, strong 92
Edam cheese 107
EGG® bread roll 118
Eggnog, regular 86
Eggplant, cooked 154
Elderberries, fresh 148
Electrolyte drink 83
Elephant ear (crispy) 118
Endive, curly, raw 154
English muffin bread 101
English muffin, whole wheat, with raisins 119
Enoki mushrooms, raw 154
Espresso, raw 92
Essentials Oat Bran cereal (Quaker®) 103
Evaporated milk, diluted, 2% fat (reduced fat) 110
Evaporated milk, skim (fat free) 92
Evaporated milk, whole 110
Extra Crispy Tenders 140

F
Falafel 136
Familia Swiss Muesli® 103
Fanta Zero®, fruit flavors 98
Fanta® Red 98
Fanta®, fruit flavors 98
Fennel bulb 154
Fennel tea 92
Feta cheese 110
Feta cheese, fat free 110
Fettuccini Alfredo®, no meat, carrots or dark green veggies 128
Fettuccini Alfredo®, no meat, vegetables except dark green 128
Fettuccini noodles 136
Fiber One Original® (General Mills®) 104
Fiber One® Nutty Clusters & Almonds (General Mills®) 104
Fifty 50® Sugar Free Butterscotch Hard Candy 123
Figs, dried, cooked, sweetened 148
Figs, fresh 148
Filberts, raw 114
Fish croquette 135
Fish or seafood with cream or white sauce 135
Fish sticks, patties / nuggets, breaded, 133
Fish with breading 133
Flax seeds, not fortified 114
Fleischmann's® Butter Margarine, tub, whipped 107
Focaccia bread 101
Fondue sauce 110
Frappuccino® 92
Frappuccino®, bottled or canned 92
Frappuccino®, bottled light 92
French Burnt Peanuts 123
French fries 138
French or Vienna roll 101
French toast 119
Froot Loops® (Kellogg's®) 104

Frosted Flakes® (Kellogg's®) 104
Frosted Flakes® Reduced Sugar (Kellogg's®) 104
Frosted Mini-Wheats Big Bite® (Kellogg's®) 104
Frozen custard, chocolate or coffee flavors 119
Frozen fruit juice Bar 160
Fruit drink or punch 95
Fruit punch, alcoholic 86
Fruit sauce, jelly-based 128

G
Garbanzo beans canned 136
Garlic, fresh 154
Gatorade®, all flavors 83
Gelatin, jello 123
German chocolate cake, glazed, homemade 119
German style potato salad, with bacon and vinegar dressing 128
GG® Scandinavian Bran Crispbread 101
Gibson 87
Gin 87
Ginger ale 98
Ginger root, raw 154
Ginko nuts, dried 115
Girl Scout® Lemonades 119
Girl Scout® Peanut Butter Patties 119
Girl Scout® Samoas® 119
Girl Scout® Shortbread® 119
Girl Scout® Thin Mints 119
Glaceau® Vitaminwater 83
Gluten free bread 101
GO Veggie!™ Rice Slices 110
Goat cheese, hard 107
GoLEAN® Crisp! Cereal, Cinnamon Crumble (Kashi®) 104
GoLEAN® Crunch! Cereal, Honey Almond Flax (Kashi®) 104
Gooseberries, fresh 148
Gorgonzola cheese 107
Gorton's® Battered Fish Fillets 133
Gorton's® Popcorn Shrimp, Original 133
Gouda cheese 107
Goulash, with beef, noodles, tomato base 133
Grand Marnier® 87
Grapefruit juice, white 95
Grapefruit, fresh, pink or red 148
Grapes, fresh 148
Grasshopper 87
Greek yogurt, plain, nonfat, 110
Green beans (string beans), cooked 154
Green bell peppers 154
Green olives 154
Green pea soup 128
Green peas, raw 136
Green tea, strong 92
Green tomato, raw 154
Grits (polenta) 154
Guava (guayaba), fresh, 148
Gum drops 123
Gum drops, sugar free 123
Gummi bears 123
Gummi bears, sugar free 123
Gummi dinosaurs 123
Gummi dinosaurs, no sugar 123
Gummi worms 123
Gummi worms, sugar free 124

H
Haagen-Dazs® Creme Brulee 160
Haagen-Dazs® Frozen Yogurt, chocolate or coffee flavors 160
Haagen-Dazs® Frozen Yogurt, vanilla or other flavors 160
Haagen-Dazs® Ice Cream, Bailey's Irish Cream 160
Haagen-Dazs® Ice Cream, Black Walnut 160
Haagen-Dazs® Ice Cream, Butter Pecan 160

Haagen-Dazs® Cherry Vanilla 160
Haagen-Dazs® Ice Cream, Chocolate 160
Haagen-Dazs® Ice Cream, Coffee 160
Haagen-Dazs® Ice Cream, Cookies & Cream 160
Haagen-Dazs® Ice Cream, Mango 160
Haagen-Dazs® Ice Cream, Pistachio 160
Haagen-Dazs® Ice Cream, Rocky Road 160
Haagen-Dazs® Ice Cream, Strawberry 161
Haagen-Dazs® Ice Cream, Vanilla Chocolate Chip 161
Half and half 110
Halvah 119
Ham croquette 135
Ham Sandwich with Veggies, no mayo 143
Hamburger 138
Hard candy 124
Hard candy, sugar free 124
Hardee's® Loaded Omelet Biscuit 128
Harvey Wallbanger 87
Health Valley® Multigrain Chewy Granola Bar, Chocolate Chip 104
Herbal tea 92
Herring, pickled 133
Hershey's® Bliss Hot Drink White Chocolate, prepared 92
Hershey's® Caramel Filled Chocolates no sugar 124
Hershey's® Milk Chocolate Bar 124
Hickorynuts 115
High-protein Bar, generic 83
Honey 104
Honey BBQ sauce 140
Honey mustard dressing 143
Honey Nut Chex® (General Mills®) 104
Honey Oat bread 143
Honey Smacks® (Kellogg's®) 104
Honeydew 148
Hot chili peppers, green, cooked 154
Hot chili peppers, red, cooked from fresh 154
Hot chocolate, homemade 92
Hot dog, combination of meats, plain 107
Hot wings 140
House side salad 140
Hubbard squash 155

I
Ice cream sandwich 161
Ice cream, light 161
Instant coffee mix, unprepared 92
Irish coffee with alcohol and whipped cream 92
Italian BMT® Sandwich with Veggies, no mayo 143

J
Jackfruit, fresh 148
Jam 107
Jam no sugar or sweetener 108
Jasmine tea 93
Jelly beans® 124
Jelly beans®, sugar free 124
Jerusalem artichoke raw 155
Jujyfruits® 124

K
Kale, raw 155
Kamikaze 87
Kashi® Chewy Granola Bar, Cherry Dark Chocolate 104
Kashi® Layered Granola Bar, Pumpkin Pecan 124
Kefir 110
Kelp, raw 155
Ken's® Apple Cider Vinaigrette dressing 138
Kern's® Mango-Orange Nectar 95
Kern's® Strawberry Nectar 95
Kidney beans, cooked from dried 155
Kirsch 87
Kit Kat® 124

Kit Kat® White 124
Kiwi fruit, gold 148
Kiwi fruit, green 148
Kohlrabi, cooked 155
Kraft® Cheese Spread, Roka Blue 108

L

Lasagna, homemade, beef 129
Lasagna, homemade, cheese, no vegetables 129
Lasagna, homemade, spinach, no meat 129
Laughing Cow® Mini Babybel®, Cheddar 110
Laughing Cow® Mini Babybel®, Original 111
Lay's® Potato Chips 115
Lay's® Potato Chips, Sour Cream & Onion 115
Lay's® Stax Potato Crisps, Cheddar 115
Lay's® Stax Potato Crisps, Hot 'n Spicy 115
Lebkuchen (German ginger bread) 119
Leeks, leafs 155
Leeks, root 155
Leeks, whole 155
Lemon juice, fresh 96
Lemon peel 162
Lemon, fresh 149
Lentil soup, condensed 129
Lentils, cooked from dried 136
Lettuce, Boston, bibb or butterhead 155
Lettuce, green leaf 155
Lettuce, iceberg 155
Lettuce, red leaf 155
Lettuce, romaine or cos 155
Libby's® Apricot Nectar 96
Libby's® Banana Nectar 96
Libby's® Juicy Juice®, Apple Grape 96
Libby's® Juicy Juice®, Grape 96
Libby's® Pear Nectar 96
Licorice 124
Licuado, mango 111
Light beer 87
Light cream 111
Lima beans, cooked from dried 155
Limburger cheese 108
Lime juice, fresh 96
Lime, fresh 149
Lipton® Iced Tea Mix, sweetened with sugar, prepared 99
Lipton® Instant 100% Tea, unsweetened, prepared 99
Liqueur, coffee flavored 87
Little Debbie® Coffee Cake, Apple Streusel 119
Little Debbie® Fudge Brownies with Walnuts 119
Little Debbie® Nutty Bars 124
Liver pudding 133
Loaf cold cut, spiced 135
Loganberries, fresh 149
Long Island iced tea 87
Long John or bismarck, glazed, cream or custard filled & nuts 119
Lotus root, cooked 156
Lowbush cranberries (lingonberries) 149
Lychees (litchis), fresh 149
Lycium (wolf or goji berries) 149
Lyonnaise (potatoes and onions) 129

M & M® cookie 143
M & M's® Peanut 124
Macadamia nuts, raw 115
Macaroni or pasta salad, with meat, egg, mayo dressing 129
Mai Tai 87
Maitake mushrooms, raw 156
Malt liquor 87
Mamba® Fruit Chews 124
Mamba® Sour Fruit Chews 124

M

Mandarin orange, fresh 149
Mango nectar 96

Mango, fresh 149
Mangosteen, fresh 149
Manhattan 87
Maple syrup, pure 104
Margarine, diet, fat free 108
Margarine, tub, salted, sunflower oil 108
Margarita, frozen 87
Marmalade, sugar free with aspartame 108
Marmalade with saccharin 108
Marmalade, sugar free with sucralose 108
Marshmallow 125
Martini® 87
Mascarpone 108
Mashed potatoes with gravy 140
McDonald's® apple slices 141
McDonald's® Barbecue sauce 141
McDonald's® Big Mac® 141
McDonald's® caramel sundae® 141
McDonald's® Cheeseburger 141
McDonald's® Chicken McNuggets® 141
McDonald's® chocolate chip cookies 141
McDonald's® chocolate milk 141
McDonald's® Crispy Chicken Snack Wrap with ranch sauce 141
McDonald's® Double Cheeseburger 141
McDonald's® Filet-O-Fish® 141
McDonald's® French fries 141
McDonald's® Hamburger 141
McDonald's® hot fudge sundae® 141
McDonald's® hot mustard 141
McDonald's® M & M McFlurry® 142
McDonald's® McCafe shakes, chocolate 142
McDonald's® McCafe shakes, vanilla or other flavors 142
McDonald's® McChicken® 142
McDonald's® McDouble® 142
McDonald's® McRib® 142
McDonald's® Newman's Own® Creamy Caesar dressing 142
McDonald's® Newman's Own® Low Fat Balsamic Vinaigrette salad dressing 142
McDonald's® orange juice 142
McDonald's® Quarter Pounder 142
McDonald's® Sausage & EGG® McMuffin® 142
McDonald's® side salad 142
McDonald's® smoothies, all flavors 142
McDonald's® Southwestern chipotle Barbecue sauce 142
McDonald's® sweet and sour sauce 142
Meat ravioli, with tomato sauce 129
Meatloaf, pork 135
Meatloaf, tuna 135
Melba Toast®, Classic (Old London®) 115
Mentos® 125
Merlot, red 87
Merlot, white 88
Milk chocolate Bar, cereal 125
Milk chocolate Bar, cereal, sugar free 125
Milk chocolate Bar, sugar free 125
Milk Chocolate covered raisins 125
Milk Maid® Caramels (Brach's®) 125
Milk, low lactose Lactaid®, skim (fat free) 111
Milk, lactose reduced Lactaid®, fortified 104
Milk, low lactose Lactaid® 93
Milk, unprepared dry powder, 93
Mineral Water 99
Minestrone soup, condensed 129

Minestrone soup, homemade 129
Mint Julep 88
Mocha, pure 93
Mojito 88
Molasses cookies, store bought 119
Molasses, dark 125
Monster® Energy® 99
Monster® Khaos 99
Morel mushrooms, raw 156
Mortadella 108
Mountain Dew® 99
Mountain Dew® Code Red 99
Mozzarella, fat free 111
Mrs. Paul's® Calamari Rings 133
Muenster cheese, natural 108
Mueslix® (Kellogg's®) 105
Muffins, banana 119
Muffins, blueberry 120
Muffins, carrot, homemade, with nuts 120
Muffins, store bought 120
Muffins, pumpkin, 120
Mulberries 149
Mung bean sprouts 156
Mung beans, cooked from dried 156
Murray® Sugar Free Oatmeal Cookies 120
Murray® Sugar Free Shortbread 120
Muscatel 88
Mushrooms, batter dipped or breaded 156
Muskmelon 149
Mustard 143

N

Nabisco® 100 Calorie Packs, Honey Maid Cinnamon Roll 120
Nectarine 149
Nestea® 100% Tea, dry 99
Nestea® Iced Tea, Sugar Free, dry 99
Nestea® Iced Tea, no sugar 99
Nestea® Iced Tea, with sugar, dry 99
Nestle® Hot Cocoa Dark Chocolate, prepared 93
Nestle® Hot Cocoa Rich Milk Chocolate 93
Nestle® Nesquik®, chocolate dry 125
Newman's Own® Organic Pretzels 101
Nilla Wafers® (Nabisco®) 120
No Fear® 99
No Fear® Sugar Free 99
Non-alcoholic wine 88
Noodle soup mix, dry 129
Northland® Cranberry Juice, all flavors 96
Nougat 125
Nutella® (filbert spread) 108
Nutter Butter® Cookies (Nabisco®) 120

O

Oat milk 111
Oatmeal cookies, store bought 120
Okra, raw 156
Old Dutch® Crunch Curls 115
Omelet, made with bacon 129
Omelet, made with sausage, potatoes, onions, cheese 129
Onion rings 138
Onion, white, yellow or red, raw 156
Oolong tea 93
Orange kiwi passion juice 96
Orange peel 162
Orange, fresh 149
Oreo® Brownie Cookies 120
Oreo® Cookies (Nabisco®) 120
Oreo® Cookies, Sugar Free 120
Oreo® Chicken Crisp® Sandwich 138
Ouzo 88
Oven Roasted Chicken Sandwich with Veggies, no mayo 143
Oyster mushrooms, raw 156

P

Pad Thai, without meat 129
Paella 129
Pancake, buckwheat 120

Pancake, whole wheat, homemade 120
Pancakes and syrup 139
Panda Express® Orange Chicken 129
Papaya, fresh 149
Parmesan cheese, dry (grated) 111
Parmesan cheese, dry (grated), nonfat 111
Parmesan Oregano bread 143
Parsnip, cooked 156
Passion fruit (maracuya), fresh 149
Passion fruit juice 96
Pasta salad with vegetables, Italian dressing 129
Peach juice 96
Peach pie, bottom crust only 120
Peach, fresh 149
Peanut butter, unsalted 115
Peanuts, dry roasted, salted 115
Pear juice 96
Pear, fresh 150
Pecan praline 125
Pepperidge Farm® Soft Sugar Cookies 121
Pepperidge Farm® Turnover, Apple 121
Pepsi® 99
Pepsi® Max 99
Pepsi® Twist 99
Persimmon, fresh 150
Pho soup (Vietnamese soup) 130
Picante taco sauce 139
Pickled beef 133
Pickled beets 156
Pillsbury® Big White Chunk Macadamia Nut Cookies 121
Pillsbury® Cinnamon Roll with Icing, all flavors 121
Pina colada 88
Pine nuts, pignolias 115
Pineapple juice 96
Pineapple orange drink 96
Pineapple, dried 150
Pineapple, fresh 150
Pistachio nuts, raw 115
Pizza Hut® cheese bread stick 130
Pizza Hut® Pepperoni Lover's pizza, stuffed crust 130
Pizza Hut® Personal Pan, supreme 130
Pizza, homemade or restaurant, cheese, thin crust 130
Plain dumplings for stew, biscuit type 136
Plantains, green, boiled 150
Plum, fresh 150
Polenta 137
Pomegranate juice 96
Pomegranate, fresh (arils-seed/juice sacs) 150
Poore Brothers® Potato Chips, Salt & Cracked Pepper 115
Popcorn, store bought (prepopped), "buttered" 121
Popsicle 161
Popsicle, sugar free 161
Pork cutlet, visible fat eaten 133
Port wine 88
Portabella mushrooms 156
Potato bread 101
Potato chips, salted 115
Potato dumpling (Kartoffelkloesse) 137
Potato gnocchi 137
Potato pancakes 137
Potato salad, with egg, mayo dressing 130
Potato soup with broccoli and cheese 130
Potato sticks 116
Potato, boiled, with skin 137
Potato, boiled, without skin 137
Power Bar® 20g Protein Plus, Chocolate Crisp 83
Power Bar® 20g Protein Plus, Chocolate Peanut Butter 83
Power Bar® 30g Protein Plus, Chocolate Brownie 84

Power Bar® Harvest Energy®, Double Chocolate Crisp 84
Power Bar® Performance Energy® 84
Powerade®, all flavors 84
Pretzels, hard, unsalted, sticks 116
Pringles® Light Fat Free Potato Crisps, Barbecue 116
Pringles® Potato Crisps, Loaded Baked Potato 116
Pringles® Potato Crisps, Original 116
Pringles® Potato Crisps, Salt & Vinegar 116
Pudding mix, other flavors, cooked type 111
Pumpernickel roll 101
Pumpkin or squash seeds 116
Purslane, raw 156

Q
Quince, fresh 150
Quinoa 137

R
Radicchio, raw 156
Radish, raw 156
Raisins, uncooked 150
Rambutan, canned in syrup 150
Ranch Crispy Chicken Wrap 139
Ranch salad dressing 144
Raspberries, fresh, red 150
Raspberry juice 97
Ratatouille 130
Red beans and rice soup mix, dry 130
Red Bull® Energy Drink 100
Red Bull® Energy Drink Sugar Free 100
Rhubarb pie, bottom crust only 121
Rhubarb, fresh 150
Ribs, beef, spare, visible fat eaten 133
Rice bread 101
Rice cake 116
Rice Krispies® (Kellogg's®) 105
Rice milk 111
Rice noodles, fried 137
Rice pudding (arroz con leche), coconut, raisins 111
Rice pudding (arroz con leche), plain 111
Rice pudding (arroz con leche), raisins 111
Ricotta cheese, part skim milk 112
Riesen® 125
Riesling 88
Ritz Cracker (Nabisco®) 116
Roast Beef Sandwich with Veggies, no mayo 144
Rob Roy 88
Rockstar Original® 100
Rockstar Original® Sugar Free 100
Rompope (eggnog with alcohol) 88
Root beer 88
Roquefort cheese 108
Rose hips 150
Rose wine, other types 88
Rum 88
Rum and cola 88
Rusty nail 88
Rutabaga, raw or blanched, marinated in oil mixture 156
Rye bread 101
Rye flour, in recipes not containing yeast 162
Rye roll 101

S
Sake 89
Salami, beer or beerwurst, beef 133
Salmon, red (sockeye), smoked 133
Sambuca 89
Sandwich cookies, vanilla 121
Sangria 89
Santa Claus melon 150
Sapodilla, fresh 150
Sauerbraten 134
Sauerkraut 157
Scallop squash 157
Scallops 134
Schnapps, all flavors 89
Schweppes® Bitter Lemon 100
Scotch and soda 89

Scrambled egg, made with bacon 130
Screwdriver 89
Sea Pak® Seasoned Shrimp, Roasted Garlic 134
Sea Pak® Shrimp Scampi in Parmesan Sauce 134
Seabreeze 89
Semolina flour 162
Sesame chicken 130
Sesame sticks 116
Shake, chocolate 139
Shake, strawberry 139
Shake, vanilla or other 139
Shallot, raw 157
Shiitake mushrooms, cooked 157
Singapore sling 89
Slim-Fast® Easy to Digest, Vanilla, ready-to-drink can 112
Sloe gin 89
Sloe gin fizz 89
Smart Balance® Light with Flax Oil Margarine, tub 108
Smart Balance® Margarine 108
Smarties® 125
Snickers® 125
Snickers®, Almond 125
Snow peas, cooked 157
Sorbet, chocolate 161
Sorbet, coconut 161
Sorbet, fruit 161
Sorghum 105
Souffle, meat 135
Soup base 130
Sour cherries, fresh 150
Sour cream 112
Sour pickles 157
Sourdough bread 101
Soursop (guanabana), fresh 151
Southern Comfort® 89
Soy bread 102
Soy chips 116
Soy Kaas Fat Free, all flavors 109
Soy milk, chocolate, sweetened with sugar, not fortified 93
Soy milk, plain or original, with artificial sweetener, ready 112
Soy milk, vanilla or other flavors, sugar, fat free, ready 112
Soybean sprouts, raw 157
Soybeans, cooked from dried 157
Spaetzle (spatzen) 137
Spaghetti squash 157
Spaghetti, with carbonara sauce 130
Spearmint tea 100
Special K® Blueberry cereal (Kellogg's®) 105
Special K® Cinnamon Pecan cereal (Kellogg's®) 105
Special K® Original cereal (Kellogg's®) 105
Special K® Red Berries cereal (Kellogg's®) 105
Spelt flour 162
Spiced ham loaf, canned 134
Spicy Italian Sandwich with Veggies, no meat 144
Spinach ravioli, with tomato sauce 130
Spinach, cooked from fresh 157
Splenda® 93
Split pea sprouts, cooked 157
Spring roll 130
Sprinkles Cookie Crisp® (General Mills®) 105
Sprite® 100
Sprite® Zero 100
Squash ravioli, with sauce 130
Starbucks® Hot Cocoa Double Chocolate 93
Starbucks® Hot Cocoa Salted Caramel, prepared 93
Starburst®, Original 126
Steak & Cheese Sandwich with Veggies 144
Stewed green peas & sofrito 131
Sticky bun 121
Stonyfield® Oikos Greek Yogurt, Blueberry 112
Stonyfield® Oikos Greek Yogurt, Caramel 112
Stonyfield® Oikos Greek Yogurt, Chocolate 112

Stonyfield® Oikos Greek Yo-gurt, Strawberry 112
Straw mushrooms, canned, drained 157
Strawberries, fresh 151
Strawberry milk, prepared 112
Strawberry pie, bottom crust only 121
Strawberry Shake 146
Streusel topping, crumb 162
Suckers®, sugar free 126
Sugar cookies, iced, store bought 121
Sugar, white granulated 126
Summer squash, cooked 157
Sunbelt Bakery® Granola Bar, Banana Harvest 105
Sunbelt Bakery® Chewy Granola Bar, Blueberry Harvest 105
Sunbelt Bakery® Chewy Granola Bar, Golden Almond 105
Sunbelt Bakery® Granola Bar, Low Fat Oatmeal Raisin 105
Sunbelt Bakery® Chewy Granola Bar, Oats & Honey 105
Sunbelt Bakery® Fudge Dipped Chewy Granola Bar, Coconut 105
Sundaes®, caramel 139
Sundaes®, chocolate fudge 139
Sundaes®, mini M & M® 139
Sundaes®, Oreo® 139
Sundaes®, strawberry 139
Sun-dried tomatoes, oil pack 157
Sunflower seeds, raw 116
Sushi, with fish 131
Sushi, with fish and vegetables in seaweed 131
Sushi, with vegetables 131
Swedish Meatballs 131
Sweet and sour chicken 131
Sweet and sour sauce 140
Sweet cherries, fresh 151
Sweet corn 140
Sweet Onion Chicken Teriyaki Sandwich with Veggies, no mayo 144
Sweet onion salad dressing 144
Sweet potato bread 121
Sweet potato, boiled 157
Sweetened condensed milk 93
Sweetened condensed milk, reduced fat 112
Swiss cheese, natural 109
Swiss cheese 109
Swiss Miss® Hot Cocoa Sensible Sweets Diet, sugar free, prepared 94
Sylvaner 89

T
Taco Bell® 7-Layer Burrito 131
Taco Bell® Beef Enchirito 145
Taco Bell® Caramel Apple Empanada 145
Taco Bell® Cheesy Fiesta Potatos 145
Taco Bell® cheesy gordita crunch 145
Taco Bell® Cinnamon Twists 145
Taco Bell® Combo Burrito 145
Taco Bell® Crunchwrap Supreme 131
Taco Bell® Double Decker Taco Supreme®, beef 145
Taco Bell® Mexican Pizza 131
Taco Bell® Nachos Supreme 131
Taco Bell® Pintos 'n Cheese 145
Taco John's® nachos 116
Taco with beans, cheese 131
Taffy 126
Tap water 100
Tempeh 157
TenderCrisp® Chicken Sandwich 139
Tequila 89
Tequila sunrise 89
Tic Tacs® 126

Tilsit cheese 109
Tiramisu 121
Toast, cinnamon and sugar, whole wheat bread 102
Toast, butter 102
Toblerone® Swiss Dark Chocolate with Honey & Almond Nougat 126
Toblerone® Swiss Milk Chocolate with Honey & Almond Nougat 126
Toblerone® Swiss White Confection with Honey & Almond Nougat 126
Toffee 126
Toffifay® 126
Tofu, raw (not silken), cooked, low fat 112
Tokaji Wine 89
Tomato juice 97
Tomato relish 131
Tomato soup mix, dry 131
Tomato, cooked from fresh 158
Tonic water 100
Tonic water, diet 100
Tootsie Pops® 126
Tortilla 116
Triple Sec 90
Triticale bread 102
Tuna Sandwich with Veggies, no mayo 144
Tuna 134
Turkey Breast & Ham Sandwich with Veggies 144
Turkey Breast Sandwich with Veggies 144
Turnip 158
Twix® 121

V
V-8® 100% A-C-E Vegetable Juice 97
Vanilla Coke® 100
Vegetable soup, condensed 131
Veggie Delite Salad 144
Veggie Delite Sandwich 144
Venison or deer, stewed 134
Veryfine Cranberry Raspberry 97
Vichyssoise 131
Vinegar 144
Vodka 90

W
Waffles, bran 121
Waffles mix 121
Walnuts 116
Watermelon, fresh 151
Wax beans 158
Weetabix® Organic Crispy 105
Wendys' 146
Werther's® Original Caramel Coffee Hard Candies 126
Wheat bran 162
Wheaties® 105
Whipped cream 94
Whipped cream, chocolate 112
Whipped cream, fat free 112
Whiskey 90
Whiskey sour 90
White flour 162
White bean stew with sofrito 131
White bread 102
White chip macadamia nut cookie 144
White chocolate Bar 126
White Russian 90
White tea 94
White whole grain wheat bread 102

White whole wheat flour 162
Whole wheat bread 102
Whopper® with cheese 139
Wild 'n Fruity Gummi Bears (Brach's®) 126
Windmill cookies 121
Wine spritzer 90
Winter melon 158
Winter type squash 158
Wise Onion Flavored Rings 116
Wrap bread 144

Y
Yams, sweet potato type 158
Yellow bell pepper, raw 158
Yellow tomato, raw 158
Yerba® Mate tea 100
Yogurt with aspartame 113
Yogurt wth sucralose 113
Yogurt, fruited, whole milk 113

Z
Zesty onion ring sauce 139
Zsweet® 126

www.ingramcontent.com/pod-product-compliance
Lightning Source LLC
Chambersburg PA
CBHW080214040426
42333CB00044B/2665